HEALTHY SHOULDER
HANDBOOK

HEALTHY SHOULDER
HANDBOOK

100
**Exercises
for Treating
and Preventing
Frozen Shoulder,
Rotator Cuff
and Other
Common Injuries**

DR. KARL KNOPF

Photography by **Austin Forbord**

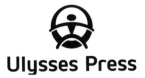

Ulysses Press

Published in the United States by Ulysses Press
P.O. Box 3440
Berkeley, CA 94703
www.ulyssespress.com

ISBN: 978-1-56975-738-3
Library of Congress Control Number 2009930128

Printed in the United States by Bang Printing

10 9 8 7

Contributing Writer	Fiona Gilbert
Acquisitions	Keith Riegert
Editorial/Production	Lily Chou, Rupa Ved, Claire Chun, Abby Reser, Lauren Harrison, Judith Metzener
Index	Sayre Van Young
Interior photos	© Austin Forbord/Rapt Productions
Illustrations	pages 13 and 14 © angelhell/istockphoto.com
Front cover design	Double R Design
Front cover photo	man © Adam Burn/gettyimages.com; woman © phildate/istockphoto.com
Back cover photos	© Austin Forbord/Rapt Productions
Models	Samuel Harvell, Scott Mathison, Meredith Miller, Bernadett Otterbein

Please Note

This book has been written and published strictly for informational purposes, and in no way should be used as a substitute for consultation with health care professionals. You should not consider educational material herein to be the practice of medicine or to replace consultation with a physician or other medical practitioner. The author and publisher are providing you with information in this work so that you can have the knowledge and can choose, at your own risk, to act on that knowledge. The author and publisher also urge all readers to be aware of their health status and to consult health care professionals before beginning any health program.

table of contents

part 1
getting
started

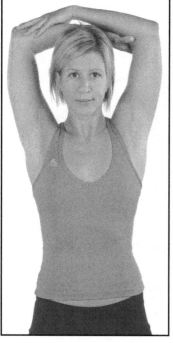

introduction

Almost everyone has a shoulder problem at some point in their lives. Most people think it won't happen to them, that it only happens to high-priced baseball pitchers or Olympic swimmers. However, approximately 14 million people visit the doctor's office each year because of a shoulder problem, although many people try to "play through" the pain—hoping it will go away—only to have a small problem become a debilitating handicap. Oftentimes, the onset of the problem manifests slowly over time and is neglected until it affects the person's range of motion or the pain is unbearable.

The incidence of shoulder dysfunction is caused by many variables. Some may result from falls, such as a tackle in football or a misstep walking down the street; others may come from overuse, such as daily golf swings or manual wheelchair use. Shoulder problems can inconvenience the weekend athlete, the office worker hunched over a computer, the home owner who paints a bedroom wall.

Here are some signs you may have a shoulder problem:

- It's difficult to move a computer mouse around on the desk.
- It hurts to reach up and put groceries away on a high shelf.
- You hear your shoulder "pop" after throwing a ball for your dog to chase or after serving an ace in tennis.
- It's uncomfortable to reach into your back pocket to grab your wallet or to reach behind your back to zip up your dress.

Most people who see the doctor for shoulder problems are affected by injuries to soft tissue surrounding the shoulder area. The goal of this book is to acquaint you with possible shoulder conditions and offer suggestions for prevention. It is not a substitute for medical care. The hope of this book is for you to learn to TRAIN SMART, NOT HARD, because learning to listen to your body and heed what it says is the wisest thing you can do. Identifying a small shoulder issue and engaging in active rest along with performing corrective exercise can go a long way in keeping you in the game.

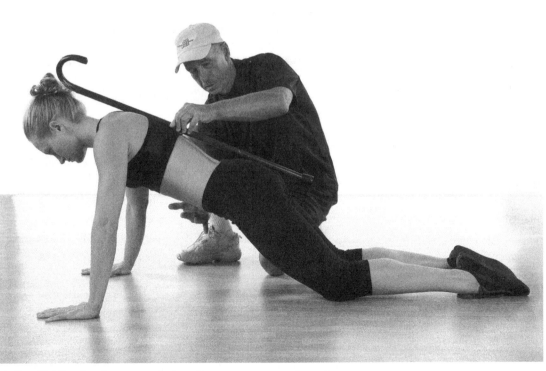

Author Karl Knopf makes some adjustments.

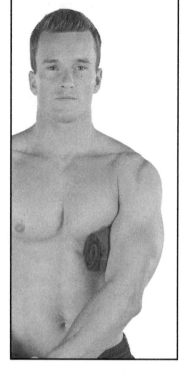

who gets shoulder problems?

The shoulder is a complex joint, and pain can be referred from the neck or other areas of the body, creating different degrees of shoulder problems. The percentage of people experiencing shoulder problems depends on the criteria used to define shoulder pain, such as pain levels or restricted movement.

Researchers compared two methods for estimating the prevalence of shoulder pain in 312 people and found that the percentage of those who had shoulder problems within the past month varied from 31 percent to 48 percent, depending on the definition of shoulder problems used. If the definition was restricted to pain rather than restricted movement, the percentage was 20 percent. However, limited range of motion—not pain—is listed as the main reason many people see their doctor.

Increasing research affirms that one body part used incorrectly can affect another body part along the kinetic chain. In simpler terms, if a person misuses his or her body biomechanically or overcompensates for a weakness in another part of the body, different parts of the body can be affected. For example, sitting incorrectly at the computer can negatively affect the shoulder, while poor hand placement on the keyboard can affect the shoulder and neck. Neck and shoulder complaints, in fact, are reported more frequently than complaints about any of the other upper body regions, and women have a higher prevalence of upper-extremity musculoskeletal complaints than men.

With regard to shoulder pain, an article in *Rehab Management* (April 2007) found that:

- Women are more often affected than men.
- People who engage in repetitive overhead motions (such as swimming the crawl or backstroke, playing tennis, washing windows or hanging wallpaper) are more prone to shoulder pain.

According to the study, a strong predictor of whether a man would get a shoulder problem in the work place depended on the type of tool used in a repetitive manner. The two predictors for women depended on if she was using a vibrating tool (the constant jarring and vibration along with the repetitive motion can lead to serious macro traumas) or if her work involved frequently keeping her arms above her head. Research found that even when women performed the same type of job at the same company as men, women had a higher incidence of shoulder complaints. With age, the prevalence increased linearly and peaked around the age of 50.

A couple of explanations have been suggested for the gender differences. Historically, women have less upper body strength than men, thus a five-pound object has a relatively greater impact on a woman, who has less strength and possibly less body weight. The European Foundation for the Improvement of Living and Working Conditions suggested that women tend to perform more repetitive work than men, and women are more likely than men to remain in a prolonged position while working. Additionally, the study found that women are often exposed to additional physical demands, such as housekeeping and childcare.

Today we see even children complaining of shoulder and neck pain. Several factors are contributing to this problem: poor posture, poor biomechanics while playing computer games, back and shoulder strain from carrying heavy backpacks, or overzealous coaches pushing children beyond their physical limits.

This book provides an overview of shoulder anatomy, as well as common causes and injuries to better understand prevention. With the supervision of your doctor, anyone can use this book to strengthen an injured shoulder or identify the onset of a shoulder problem.

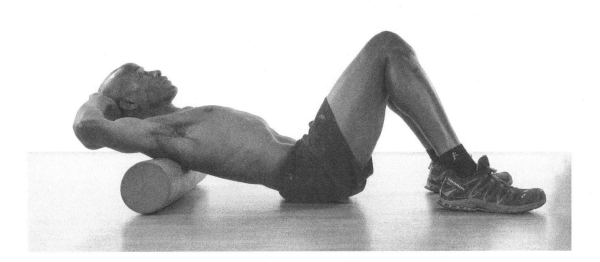

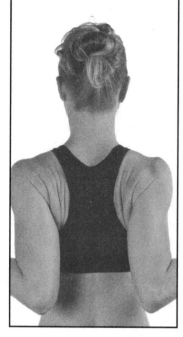

shoulder anatomy

The shoulder, more accurately called the "shoulder girdle," is a remarkable, complex joint. It can gently toss an egg back and forth, rock a baby to sleep, hurl a baseball at 90 mph and generate a 100-mph serve in tennis. An engineering marvel, its design allows for maximum flexibility and function in almost every conceivable direction.

This mobility, however, is also why the shoulder joint is so vulnerable to overuse and injuries, and one reason why it is the most difficult and complicated joint in the body to rehabilitate.

To understand and commit to the rehabilitation process, you need to have a basic understanding of the shoulder joint and its kinesiology. By understanding your condition, you'll better understand the steps needed to fully recover.

The shoulder joint consists of a large ball and smaller socket. The basic structure is similar to a sideways-lying golf tee with a tennis ball next to it, held in place with a series of bands called ligaments and tendons. Ligaments attach bone to bone while tendons attach muscle to bone. This anatomical design, unfortunately, does not provide a great deal of structural support. Generally, in the human body, extensive flexibility at a joint also means reduced stability. By comparison, the hip is also a ball and socket joint, but it's a deep socket, which provides a great deal of structural support but not much mobility. The shoulder joint's ligaments and tendons impart stability, but these bands can become lax through misuse and chronic overuse.

Bones and Joints

The shoulder girdle is composed of four bones. The *clavicle* is commonly known as the collar bone. The *scapula* is also known as the shoulder blades, or wing/angel bones; the *acromion* is the part of the scapula that forms a bony roof above the rotator cuff, tendons and bursa. The *sternum* is often referred to as the breast bone. The *humerus* is the upper bone of the arm.

Joints, where bones come together, are surrounded by soft tissue, which includes ligaments, tendons and bursas. There are several joints/articulations of the shoulder. The majority of the joint movement occurs in the GH joint; the other joints serve more as supporting structures.

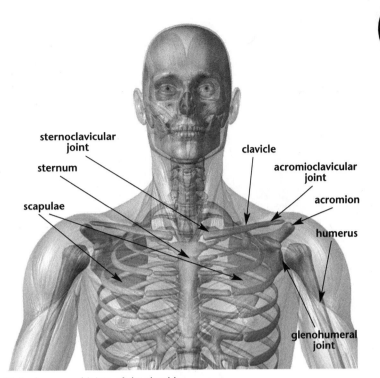

Major bones and joints of the shoulder

- **Acromioclavicular (AC)**—This joint is formed by the acromion and the clavicle. Mainly, it is active with shrugging movements.
- **Glenohumeral (GH)**—The combination of the upper arm bone and the outside area of the scapula makes up this joint. This joint is responsible for most of the movements of the shoulder. Shoulder dislocation always refers to this joint.
- **Sternoclavicular (SC)**—This joint is composed of the clavicle and the sternum. This joint primarily operates during shrugs, although part of its function is to stabilize the shoulder girdle.

- **Scapulothoracic (ST)**—This is not really a moveable joint but serves as a base for muscles to be secured to.

Each of the four rotary cuff muscles (see "Muscles" below) originates on the scapula and their tendons attach to the top of the humerus, helping to form the joint capsule. The sac surrounding the joint is called a bursa. A fluid-filled bursa is usually found between bones and tendons to help decrease friction during normal joint use. It provides lubrication to the joint. Cartilage is the gristle/pad between joints, providing cushion to the joint.

Muscles

Before we move on to the muscles of the shoulder, remember that muscles can do two things: contract or relax. Agonist muscles are responsible for contraction movements, while antagonist muscles produce an action opposite of the agonist. In addition, stabilizers anchor or support a bone so the agonist can have a firm base from which to operate.

The following make up the major muscles of the shoulder.

- **Supraspinatus** abducts the arm (i.e., moves the arm away from the body).
- **Infraspinatus** rotates the arm laterally.

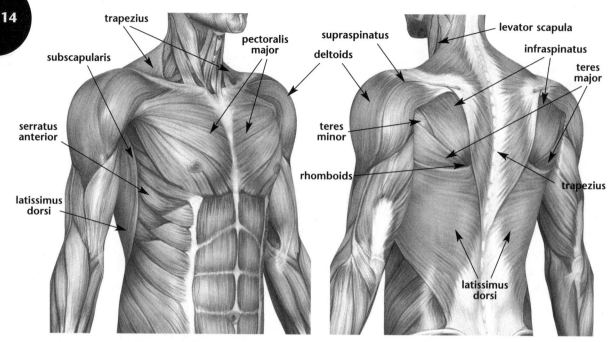

Major muscles that affect the shoulder

- **Teres minor** rotates the arm laterally.
- **Teres major** adducts the arm (i.e., brings the arm in to the body).
- **Subscapularis** internally rotates the arm.
- **Latissimus dorsi** extends and adducts the arm.
- **Trapezius** elevates and depresses the scapula.
- **Pectoralis major & minor** adducts the arm and pulls the scapula downward.

- **Coracobrachialis** flexes and adducts the arm.
- **Deltoid** abducts and extends the arm.
- **Levator scapula** moves the neck laterally.
- **Rhomboid major & minor** stabilizes the scapula.
- **Serratus anterior** stabilizes the scapula.

Other than trauma and repetitive chronic misuses, muscle imbalances, whether caused by work duties or recreational activities, are the prime culprit when it comes to shoulder injury. If one set of muscles gets too tight, the delicate balance of the space in the shoulder complex is upset, possibly throwing the alignment out of place. This is similar to the guide wires of a radio tower; if they're too tight, they can cause a misalignment. These misalignments set the stage for injury.

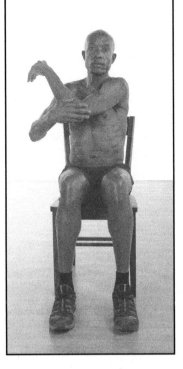

common shoulder conditions

As with most joint conditions, shoulder problems can be traced back to misuse, overuse, disuse or abuse of shoulder muscles. Anything that affects any part of the kinetic chain can cause problems. For instance, taking a bad fall (abuse) or painting the ceiling for two hours straight (misuse/ overuse) may result in an unhappy shoulder.

Unfortunately, age does play a factor in shoulder conditions. As we age, the soft tissues surrounding the shoulder girdle undergo some structural changes. Often, these structural changes lead to the weakening of the supporting ligaments, tendons and muscles. Some experts in the field suggest that by 50 years of age, most people have some internal shoulder structural changes. Often, a simple tendinitis can degenerate into

actual tearing of the muscle tissues. If simple tendinitis is not properly treated, further episodes can lead to greater damage—which is why early intervention and preventative maintenance is the key to complete shoulder health. (The section on injury prevention starts on page 30.)

This section provides an overview of common shoulder conditions and includes typical causes, symptoms and treatments. Unless you're an

expert on shoulders, it is *always* recommended that you consult your doctor for an accurate diagnosis. When you speak with the doctor, he or she will often take a health history and do a physical exam to make a diagnosis.

A highly regarded assessment tool is the subjective shoulder scale assessment used with rotator cuff, shoulder instability and arthritis clients. When given this assessment, you'll be evaluated on whether you experience difficulty putting on a coat, sleeping on your side, reaching behind you, combing your hair, reaching a high shelf, throwing a ball overhand, or performing work duties or recreational pursuits.

Shoulder Impingement

Shoulder impingement is a somewhat common chronic condition seen in people who are extremely hypermobile. That extra flexibility leads to repetitive stress and inflammation.

Symptoms

- Pinching sensation when raising arm
- Pain when sleeping on one side
- Pain accompanies arm movement

Common Causes

Shoulder impingement can be caused by repetitive activity that requires the shoulder joint to do overhead motions day in and day out, such as:

- Tennis
- Swimming
- Throwing sports, such as baseball and softball
- Excessive overhead arm motions: working in a warehouse, home repairs
- Sleeping on the same arm each night
- Trauma, such as falling on shoulder

Assessment

- Range-of-motion tests
- A simple assessment of muscle imbalances and muscle testing wherein the health practitioner uses manual resistance to compare the weakness of the client's affected side against the non-affected side
- X-ray or MRI

Treatment

The doctor may offer you many options, ranging from rest, learning to use your shoulder more biomechanically correctly, physical therapy modalities, corrective exercises, injections and surgery.

The therapist or doctor may also:

- Instruct you how to use heat and ice.
- Recommend medication and medicated pads.
- Apply electrical stimulation or ultrasound treatments.
- Suggest steroid injections in the joint area.

Repetitive Motion Injuries (RMI), a.k.a. Cumulative Trauma Disorder

Using the same arm over and over again can aggravate your tendons, ligaments, bursa sac or cartilage.

Symptoms

- Pain in shoulder, hand or arm when lying on that side of the body
- Numbness in arm or fingers
- Tingling in hands, arm or fingers
- Chronic aching in shoulder or arm

Common Causes

- Repetitive overhead motion
- Repetitive use of forceful movement

Assessment

Generally, the health practitioner will take you through a series of movements with and without resistance to evaluate the specific issues you have. The most important thing you can do to expedite the exam is to specify which movements bring the most discomfort. The health practitioner will also ask you if the pain comes on suddenly and which activities make it worse.

Treatment

The doctor may prescribe medications, splints, physical therapy and possible surgery or injections, depending on the severity of your condition.

Shoulder Instability (Dislocation/Subluxation)

Due to its design, the shoulder joint is one of the most frequently dislocated joints of the body. The dislocation often results from a strong force that pulls the shoulder/arm outward or through an extreme rotation that "pops" the ball (the head of the humerus) out of the joint. Note that partial dislocations are possible. In a subluxation, the shoulder feels like it slipped out of the socket and then slipped back into place without a complete separation. Having a complete separation/dislocation is far more damaging and, once a shoulder dislocates, dislocations can occur more frequently.

Symptoms

The arm is physically out of the joint, making it impossible to move the arm. There is also moderate pain.

Common Causes

- Falling
- Running into something/someone
- Lifting incorrectly
- Reaching past your safety zone

Assessment

The health practitioner will look at the joint and see if it's displaced. He or she will also determine whether or not you're able to move the arm.

Treatment

If you suspect you have any level of separation of the shoulder joint, IMMEDIATELY go to a trained professional to have it repositioned. Once the joint has been re-positioned, follow the doctor's orders and an exercise routine to improve the stability of the joint.

Arthritis

Osteoarthritis of the shoulder is a degenerative condition in which the cartilage deteriorates. This is often the result of chronic wear and tear. However, it can be caused by disease, trauma or infection. Arthritis of the shoulder is seen in the AC joint earlier than the GH joint because the AC joint degenerates more quickly.

Symptoms

Mild to moderate pain in the shoulder area and limited range of motion.

Common Causes

- Wear and tear
- Rheumatoid arthritis
- Trauma
- Muscle imbalances
- Poor body mechanics when exercising, such as during deep bench presses and dips
- Overtraining

Assessment

A doctor will conduct a health history and a physical evaluation asking you to perform a range of simple motions.

Treatment

- Rest
- NSAIDs
- Injections
- Physical therapy

Rotator Cuff Injuries

Some experts believe that when you move your arm, as many as 26 muscles are engaged in the movement phase, the stabilization phase or the deceleration phase. At the gym, people often focus only on the superficial, visible muscles while neglecting crucial, deep muscles that support and provide stabilization to the joint. The rotator cuff is made up of the SITS muscles: Subscapularis, Infraspinatus, Teres minor and Supraspinatus. These muscles share a common tendon. The rotator cuff is responsible for internal and external rotation most commonly seen in throwing a ball or serving a tennis ball.

It was once thought that rotator cuff injuries were the result of sudden or severe trauma. It is now believed that degenerative changes occur over time as the result of misuse or abuse or may also be brought on by trauma.

Symptoms

- Overhead motions (such as reaching for something on a high shelf, combing

SAMPLE ROTATOR CUFF PROGRAM

your hair, and throwing a ball) cause pain.

- It hurts to scratch your mid-back.
- It hurts to sleep on your shoulder.

Common Causes

Repetitive use and trauma are the most common mechanisms of a rotator cuff injury. Rotator cuff tears are seen quite often between the ages of 45 and 65. The most familiar repetitive injuries include poor execution of exercises in the weight room, lat pulls behind the neck or improper bench presses (see page 35 for common controversial exercises), and overuse with throwing sports. Rotator cuff injuries are also often the result of:

- Overuse tendinitis: Leads to irritation and fraying of the tendon
- Impingement tendinitis: The acromion can pinch and irritate the rotator cuff, or the bursa is swollen as a result of repetitive overhead motion.
- Calcification tendinitis: Inflammation can lead to calcium deposits within the rotator cuff.
- Severe tendinitis: Tears can cause partial or complete tearing of the rotator cuff.

Assessment

During your assessment, your doctor will take a health history, asking many questions about when your shoulder hurts and how you think you hurt it. Your doctor will perform a physical exam looking for signs of weakness, and he or she will listen for popping and grinding sounds. Often, the doctor will have you do the "soda can test," which is done by moving your arm as if pouring out soda. The doctor will gently resist the motion to determine the extent of the injury.

If a diagnosis cannot be made from the physical exam, the doctor may order imaging tests such as MRIs, x-rays and arthrograms (dye is injected into the shoulder for this procedure).

Treatment

Generally, most doctors will try conservative care of rest, cold and heat packs, and medication. If that does not work, you may be referred to physical therapy, where corrective exercises along with ultrasound (gentle sound-wave vibrations) and electrical stimulation treatments may be administered. Some doctors will use cortisone injections to reduce the inflammation. If these fail to bring relief, surgical options may be discussed.

Frozen Shoulder

Your shoulder is designed to move freely in many directions. When pain limits your movement, you'll generally reduce your range of motion. This allows adhesions to develop, and your shoulder "freezes." As these adhesions develop, they make movement even more difficult and painful—leading to further reduction of motion and a more frozen shoulder. This cycle of disuse sets up increased pain and immobility. Women are more likely to manifest a frozen shoulder than men. This is often a result of an injury or the consequence of an attempt to protect the shoulder. It is seen more often in older people than younger.

Symptoms

- Pain in all directions
- Reduced range of motion

Common Causes

When a person experiences shoulder pain, he or she tries to protect the joint by not moving it. This leads to inflammation as well as the development of adhesive capulitis, where the shoulder capsule adheres to the head of the humerus.

Assessment

During your assessment, your doctor will take a health history and conduct a physical exam.

Treatment

The objective is to increase motion and reduce pain. Your doctor may engage in aggressive joint mobilizations along with stretching and electrical stimulation. He or she may also suggest the following options to treat your frozen shoulder:

- Shoulder stretches
- Anti-inflammatory medications
- Mild and moist heat
- Ice applications
- Physical therapy or manual therapy and modalities
- Cortisone injections
- Surgical interventions

Tendinitis and Bursitis

Tendinitis and bursitis are closely related and may occur alone or in combination. *Tendinitis* is inflammation (redness, soreness, swelling) of a tendon. In tendinitis of the shoulder, the rotator cuff and/or biceps tendon become inflamed, usually as a result of being pinched by surrounding structures. The injury may vary from mild inflammation to involvement of most of the rotator cuff. When the rotator cuff tendon becomes inflamed and thickened, it may get trapped beneath the acromion. Tendinitis is often accompanied by inflammation of the bursa sacs that protect the shoulder. An inflamed bursa is called *bursitis*.

Symptoms

Signs of these conditions include:

- The slow onset of discomfort and pain in the upper shoulder or upper third of the arm.
- Difficulty sleeping on the shoulder.
- Pain when the arm is lifted away from the body or overhead. If tendinitis involves the biceps tendon (the tendon located in front of the shoulder that helps bend the elbow and turn the forearm), pain will occur in the front or side of the shoulder and may travel down to the elbow and forearm.
- Pain when the arm is forcefully pushed upward overhead.

Common Causes

When the rotator cuff and bursa are irritated, inflamed and swollen, they may become squeezed between the head of the humerus and the acromion. Repeated motion involving the arms, or simply the aging process, may also irritate and wear down the tendons, muscles and surrounding structures. Inflammation resulting from a disease such as rheumatoid arthritis may cause rotator cuff tendinitis and bursitis. Sports that overuse the shoulder and occupations requiring frequent overhead reaching are other potential causes of irritation to the rotator cuff or bursa, and may lead to inflammation.

Assessment

Diagnosis of tendinitis and bursitis begins with a medical history and physical examination. X-rays do not show tendons or the bursa, but they may be helpful in ruling out bony abnormalities or arthritis. The doctor may remove and test fluid from the inflamed area to rule out infection.

Treatment

The majority of patients who see their doctor about a shoulder problem are there because of tendinitis. Most cases of tendinitis can be successfully treated. The first step in treating these conditions is to reduce pain and inflammation with rest, ice and anti-inflammatory medicines such as aspirin, naproxen or ibuprofen (e.g., Advil, Motrin or Nuprin). In some cases, the doctor or therapist will use ultrasound to warm deep tissues and improve blood flow. Before self-medicating, consult your doctor. Also, don't medicate yourself to cover up the pain so you can continue to play or work. While you may feel fine, you can be damaging the joint.

Gentle stretching and strengthening exercises are recommended and gradually added as you improve. The therapist may suggest applying a warm pack and engaging in gentle active motion followed by an ice pack. If there is no improvement, the doctor may inject a corticosteroid medicine into the space under the acromion. While steroid injec-

tions are a common treatment, they must be used with caution because they can lead to tendon rupture. If there is still no improvement after 6 to 12 months, the doctor may perform either arthroscopic or open surgery to repair damage and relieve pressure on the tendons and bursae.

Thoracic Outlet Syndrome (TOS)

Thoracic Outlet Syndrome, while not very common, is often misunderstood and misdiagnosed. The term "TOS" first appeared in medical literature in 1956 in an article published by R. M. Peet and colleagues entitled "Thoracic Outlet Syndrome." TOS has been the subject of much controversy, and some experts have expressed that it is one of the most poorly understood, under-diagnosed and misdiagnosed conditions.

TOS may be loosely defined as a group of disorders producing a constellation of signs and symptoms due to compression of blood vessels and nerves (neurovascular bundle) in the thoracic outlet region. The thoracic outlet is a space located between the rib cage (thorax) and the clavicle, which contains major blood vessels (subclavian artery and

vein) and nerves (brachial plexus).

Since some experts believe that TOS is under-diagnosed, and in some cases misdiagnosed, it is difficult to estimate with any degree of accuracy how many people suffer from this condition. The incidence of TOS in the U.S. population has been broadly estimated to range from 0.3 percent to 8 percent. The most common age range is 25 to 40 years, and women are affected about four times more frequently than men.

As mentioned above, TOS is not a single disorder but rather a group of distinct disorders that produce signs/symptoms suggestive of compression or pressure of the blood vessels and/or nerves in the thoracic outlet region. For example, symptoms such as a pain in the neck/shoulder/arms and a sense of numbness or tingling suggest a compression of the nerves of the brachial plexus; weakness, swelling or coldness in the arm/hand may be caused by a compression of the subclavian blood vessels, resulting in decreased blood flow to the area. In general, the various groups of TOS may be classified as follows:

True neurogenic TOS: This type of TOS is also called neurologic TOS and is a rare disorder caused by congenital (birth) anomalies (cervical rib and band syndrome). It usually affects one side of the body and predominantly occurs in women ages 15 to 60 years. Symptoms include weakness and atrophy of the hand, primarily involving the arm muscles and intermittent aching, numbness and parasthesia (burning or tingling sensation), which may also involve the fingers or arms. True neurogenic TOS may often be confused with carpal tunnel syndrome.

Traumatic TOS: As the name implies, this type of TOS occurs following trauma or injury. The most common type of trauma involves a fracture of the clavicle (collar bone), which may also cause secondary injury to the nerves and blood vessels within the thoracic outlet. Traumatic TOS usually develops on the same side where the injury has occurred. The most frequent symptom is pain in the neck/shoulder area, which may be accompanied by weakness and/or numbness in the arm/hand.

Disputed TOS: This category of TOS is by far the most common type seen by doctors. The term "disputed TOS" (also known as non-specific TOS)

was applied to this disorder because its existence is controversial. While some experts believe that it is a real disorder and occurs frequently, others have argued that it does not exist as a true clinical condition. The most prominent symptoms of disputed TOS include pain, parasthesia and weakness. However, extensive clinical examination often fails to detect any objective evidence of an underlying problem of cause, which is why some experts have argued that this disorder does not exist. Several theories have been proposed regarding the underlying cause of disputed TOS including trauma to the brachial plexus, congenital anomalies or postural abnormalities.

True Vascular TOS: This type of TOS involves damage to the subclavian artery or vein and can be documented by performing an arteriogram or venogram, which demonstrates reduced blood flow to the area. Symptoms may include pain, numbness and coldness in the hands and fingers, as well as the presence of sores on the fingers. True vascular TOS is a rare disorder and may be caused by a congenital anomaly.

Symptoms
- Pain in the neck/shoulder arms and a sense of numbness or tingling
- Weakness, swelling or coldness in the arm/hand
- Neck/shoulder pain that may spread to the upper arm and forearm
- Pain that radiates down the arm
- Numbness/weakness along the forearm, hand and pinky
- Headaches involving the occipital or orbital areas
- Anterior chest wall pain (pseudo-angina)
- Swelling of the arm/hand
- Coldness in the hand/fingers
- Blue color of the hand/fingers
- Wasting (atrophy) of the hand (in severe, chronic cases of TOS)

Common Causes
- Studies have shown that TOS is associated with jobs that incorporate heavy lifting (e.g., jackhammer operators, electricians, carpenters), as well as certain occupations that involve working in a static position for an extended period of time (e.g., secretaries, computer operators, benchworkers).

Both of these contribute to postural abnormalities.

- Trauma such as clavicle fractures, trauma to the shoulder, hyperextension injuries of the neck (whiplash)
- Congenital anomalies (cervical rib and band syndrome), abnormal fibromuscular bands present at birth that irritate or compress the brachial plexus
- Postural distortions such as drooping or sagging shoulders

Assessment

The following conditions, which produce signs and symptoms that may be confused with TOS, must be ruled out before a diagnosis of TOS can be considered:

- Carpal tunnel syndrome
- Cervical spine disease with nerve root compression
- Pancoast tumor (a type of lung tumor that grows in the thoracic inlet)
- Spinal cord tumor
- Degenerative spinal cord diseases (e.g., multiple sclerosis, syringomyelia)
- Other neuropathies (e.g., cubital tunnel syndrome, radial runnel compression)

- Tumor of the brachial plexus
- Inflammatory diseases of the shoulder (e.g., tendinitis, arthritis)
- Complex regional pain syndrome (e.g., reflex sympathetic dystrophy [RSD])
- Vascular diseases (e.g., atherosclerosis, thrombophlebitis)

A variety of diagnostic tests may be used in assessing patients with signs and symptoms of TOS. None of these tests are specific for TOS—they're used primarily to rule out other possible causes of symptoms that the patient experiences.

- Chest x-ray
- MRI of cervical spine
- CT scan of the brachial plexus
- Electromyography test used to measure muscle response to stimulation of nerves
- Nerve conduction studies
- Angiography of venography, if blood flow problems are suspected

Treatment

The objectives of treatment for patients with TOS include relieving and eliminating compression of the nerves and/or blood vessels in the thoracic outlet region; controlling and minimizing pain and other signs and symptoms associated with TOS; and improving the patient's overall quality of life. Most experts agree that a conservative approach is the first round of treatment in the management of patients with TOS unless the patient is experiencing significant neurologic impairment or acute vascular insufficiency due to neurovascular compression; in this case, surgery may be necessary. Approximately 85 percent of patients with TOS will improve with conservative treatment and only a small percentage of patients actually require surgery.

- Physical therapy
- Muscle-strengthening exercises
- Stretching/isometric exercises
- Postural training to correct poor posture (drooping or sagging shoulders)
- Osteopathic manipulation of the scalene and trapezius muscles
- Heat treatments with ultrasound
- Transcutaneous Electrical Nerve Stimulation (TENS) to control pain

- Swimming, although some authorities recommend avoiding the backstroke and breaststroke
- Drug therapy
- Analgesics and non-steroidal anti-inflammatory drugs (NSAIDs) to reduce pain and inflammation
- Muscle relaxants to control muscle spasms
- Antidepressants may be necessary for TOS patients with comorbid depression
- Scalene injections with local anesthetic/steroid solutions to reduce pain
- Stellate ganglion block may be given to patients with TOS who also have symptoms of RSD
- Surgery

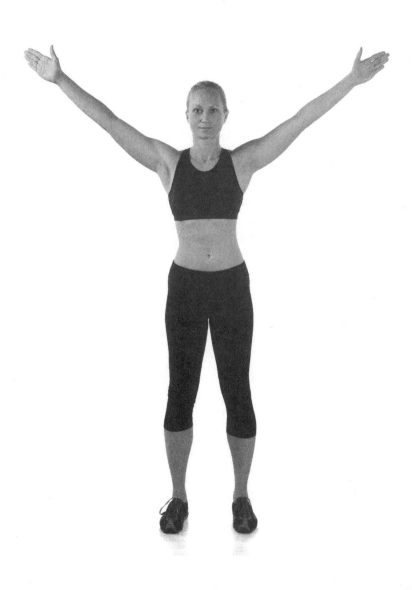

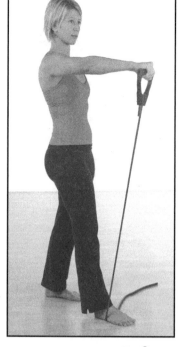

shoulder rehab

You can greatly improve your chances of a full and rapid recovery by promptly visiting your doctor upon feeling pain, especially if you suffer from numbness in the hands and fingers or experience severe loss of function. Before starting any type of rehabilitation, have a doctor or therapist perform a complete evaluation of both your active range of motion (your ability to move your joint on your own) and passive range of motion (the ability of your health provider to move your joint).

During the examination, the health provider will compare the affected side to the non-affected side and evaluate the source, cause and level of the shoulder pain as well as the range of motion and function. He or she will also perform a muscle test to ascertain which muscles are involved. The health provider may order a further exam, such as an MRI, before determining a course of therapy.

After a medical examination, you'll be given a diagnosis, which will indicate affected areas and the severity of injury.

The three general classifications of injury are:

MILD—At this stage, the doctor may recommend a home-based exercise program that includes corrective exercise and specific stretches. Keep in mind, you are still injured and re-injury is very

common. Do not rush the body's healing.

MODERATE—At this stage, passive and light active range-of-motion exercises may be advised to prevent a frozen shoulder. Protective rest of the joint, as well as modalities to control pain, will be recommended.

SEVERE—At this stage, rest, ice and heat applications and range of motion exercises are often recommended. Pain-

Knowing the cause of an injury is critical in developing a comprehensive rehabilitation program. Some injuries are the result of a sudden impact; others are the result of chronic misuse, overuse and abuse of the body or body parts. Generally speaking, there are two types of injury, macro trauma and micro trauma.

Macro trauma is an injury due to a specific event. The time, place and mechanism of injury are usually quite clear. The single event results in a previously normal/healthy structure becoming suddenly and distinctly abnormal after the event (e.g., shoulder separation).

Micro traumas are chronic, repetitive injuries. These injuries actually arise from misalignments and poor body mechanics combined with repetitive insults to the area. Chronic conditions, unlike acute injuries, must be managed and cannot be quickly resolved.

management options such as medications or possible injections can be discussed.

Preventing further damage is critical. Attempting to "play through" pain and dismissing your injury will only prolong the rehabilitation process. Avoid movements such as overhead motions, sleeping on your affected side or hanging your bag over your affected shoulder. Restoration of shoulder function should address both the local and general effects of the injury and comprehensively treat both the injury and the total person. Note that muscle strength can decrease up to 17 percent within the initial 72 hours of immobilization. The rate of decline slows after five to seven days, but muscle strength loss of up to 40 percent has been seen after six weeks of immobilization. The longer the immobilization period, the greater chance of soft tissue dysfunction and muscle atrophy, thus causing prolonged rehabilitation.

Note that the absence of symptoms does not mean full restoration. Just treating the injury and neglecting the total person will set the individual up for another injury. In athletes, 30 to 50 percent of all sports injuries are related to overuse or improper training techniques. Some studies have shown that 27 percent of these injuries are re-injuries, and that 16 percent occurred within one month of returning to play.

Also, remember the two-hour rule: If you hurt more than two hours after an exercise session, you need to reduce activity to a level that does not cause pain; if you continue to hurt or lose range of motion, consult your doctor ASAP. An effective rehabilitation routine will train both the brain and the body, which is why you need to be mindful when training. In today's managed health care, physical therapists often don't have time to fully attend to all the aspects needed for complete restoration. This is why *you* play a significant part in restoring yourself to full function.

The Therapy Process

Once an accurate diagnosis is made, your therapist will design a treatment plan for your specific condition. The therapist will guide you along the steps, with your pain level and range of motion being key criteria for how much you should or shouldn't do.

It's important to keep in mind that each person has his or her own timetable for recovery, and that the absence of pain is not a sign to return to "normal" activity. Also, many times people develop compensatory adjustments to make up for functional deficits, which may lead to further dysfunction. Justifying compensatory movements is generally not acceptable as these movements might only cause trauma further up or down the kinetic chain.

The rehabilitation goals occur in three stages: acute, recovery and function.

Phase 1: Acute Stage

The acute stage focuses on preventing further harm, decreasing the signs and symptoms of injury, and hastening the healing process. A trained therapist should oversee this phase of rehabilitation.

The goals of Phase 1 are to:
- Manage pain
- Maintain range of motion
- Maintain neuromuscular control
- Prevent muscle atrophy.

The criteria for advancement to phase 2 are:

- Pain control
- Healing tissue
- Near-normal range of motion
- Tolerance for strength training.

Phase 2: Recovery Phase

This phase can be done with an adaptive fitness personal trainer or by yourself—as long as you/he/she stays within the scope of practice and is following the protocols set forth by the medical professional. At this stage, many people re-injure themselves, so be careful.

The goals of Phase 2 are to:
- Prevent further injury and pain
- Regain upper body strength and muscular balance and stability
- Foster shoulder flexibility
- Improve neuromuscular control and coordination
- Be evaluated for progression to next level.

The criteria for advancement to phase 3 are:
- No pain
- Complete tissue healing
- Almost complete range of motion
- Near-normal strength when compared to the uninvolved side (approximately 75 to 80 percent).

Phase 3: Function Phase

This phase can be done with an adaptive fitness personal trainer or by yourself—as long as you/he/she stays within the scope of practice and is following the protocols set forth by the medical professional. Once you've re-gained full functional recovery, evaluate the circumstances that may have caused your condition and adapt your lifestyle and behaviors. By being sensible, following your therapist's suggestions and participating in the exercises included in this book, you reduce your chances of re-injuring yourself.

The goals of Phase 3 are to:
- Learn the importance of proper training techniques
- Learn how to exercise the stabilizing muscles and learn proper posture and lifestyle changes to prevent future injury
- Increase muscular strength and endurance in preparation for work or sports demands
- Improve multi-plane range of motion
- Institute sport-specific drills and functional activities of daily living
- Be evaluated to see if you are ready to re-engage in a fully active lifestyle.

The criteria for knowing you've reached "full functional recovery" are:

- Zero pain
- Full and complete pain-free range of motion/flexibility
- Strength equal to the uninvolved side
- Normal body mechanics.

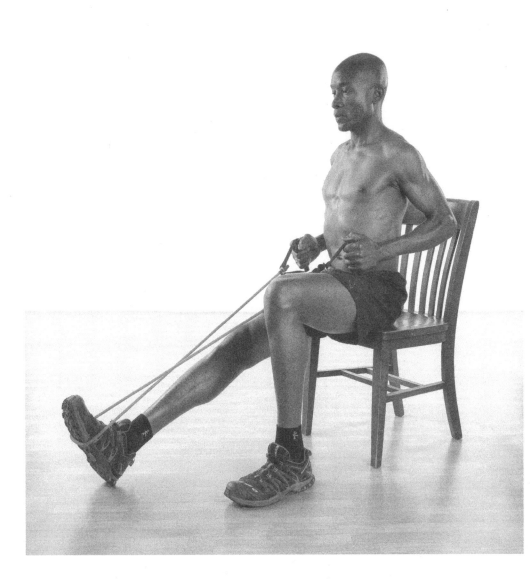

part 2

prevention & programs

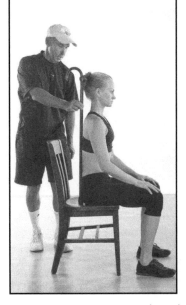

preventing (re)injury

We're all familiar with the saying "An ounce of prevention is worth a pound of cure." We all understand that preventing a problem is a wise idea. This concept is relevant in protecting our shoulder joint just as it is in maintaining our automobile, whether it's a regular oil change or tune-up. Preventive maintenance can prevent a breakdown or an expensive repair. Unfortunately, when it comes to our bodies, we oftentimes neglect that basic idea.

Let's assume you've recovered from a shoulder injury, or are on your way to full function. Staying proactive provides the best defense against a recurring shoulder problem. One way you can prevent a shoulder problem is by asking your doctor how to best use heat and ice. Most therapists suggest moist heat to loosen a joint, followed by active warm-up to foster improved range of motion, followed by ice after activity.

You should also begin a comprehensive shoulder conditioning program with a specific stretching routine. While strength training is a good thing, too much can cause too much tightness and possible injury. While stretching is good, too much can lead to a lax joint and possible re-injury. Remember: More is not always better! Joseph Pilates (the father of Pilates exercises) said it best, "Stretch what is tight, strengthen what is lax."

The exercises in Part 3 of this book have been selected from a review of the best therapeutic exercise publications addressing the shoulder. Treat this book as a menu from which you (either in consultation with your health professional or simple experimentation) select appropriate exercises for your condition. If you've had physical therapy, you might even recognize some of these exercises. The exercises in this book can be done in a proactive manner, but if you notice that you're manifesting some shoulder concerns, it's always wise to talk to your health provider. Otherwise, start with the most gentle exercise and progress from there.

Here are some basic guidelines to follow when determining which exercises to do. If in doubt, consult with your health provider.

If you've had chronic/recurrent shoulder instabilities, ask your health provider if you can do:

- Isometric exercises to increase internal and external muscles
- Resistance tubing exercises.

(You may need to wear a protective device to limit your shoulder motions.)

If you've experienced shoulder impingement, you should:

- Re-learn proper body mechanics.
- Strengthen rotator cuff muscles.
- Strengthen lower extremities to reduce shoulder strain when throwing.

(Be alert to what caused the incident and be careful. If you're over 40, be especially mindful. Use RICE—rest, ice, compression, elevation—when needed.)

If you've had bursitis, you should:

- Avoid overuse.
- Maintain flexibility.

If you have arthritis, you should:

- Avoid overuse.
- Balance strengthening exercises with flexibility exercises.

You'll also find sample programs for common activities starting on page 43.

Posture's Role in Prevention

Most people know that poor posture can lead to back pain, but posture also plays an important role in shoulder health. For instance, the rounded-shoulder, forward-head posture (think turtle) is often seen in people who swim a lot using the crawl/freestyle stroke without strengthening the opposing

muscle group and stretching the chest muscles. This decreased flexibility of the chest and shoulder can set the stage for shoulder problems. Experts now understand that if one body part is misaligned, overused or hurt, it can affect the mechanics somewhere along the kinetic chain.

Look for the image of good posture below. Notice that her ear, shoulder, hip and ankle are all on the same vertical line. Any deviation from this alignment can lead to a multitude of issues, from neck and shoulder problems to low back pain. Of course, plenty of things, like working a desk job, sitting in a cramped airplane seat, and fixing a car, will challenge your ability to maintain good posture. That's why you should assess your

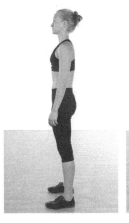

Good posture: ear, shoulder, hip and ankle are all on the same vertical line

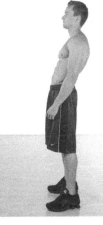

Poor posture: Excessive arch of the lower back (lordosis)

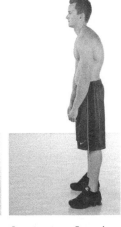

Poor posture: Excessive roundness of the upper back (kyphosis)

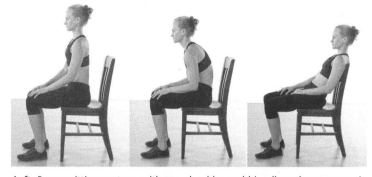

Left: *Proper sitting posture, with ear, shoulder and hip all on the same verti-cal line.* **Midde and right:** *Poor sitting posture.*

posture several times a day.

The easiest way to do this is to stand with your back against a wall, with your heels no more than 6 inches from the wall. Place your bottom to the wall then attempt to place your upper back and the base of your head to the wall, keeping your chin down. If you have very compromised posture, start with just placing your bottom against the wall; as you improve, take your time trying to get your upper back against the wall before finally attempting to get your head to the wall. Some older people with severely compromised posture never get their head to the wall, so start today before it's too late. Practicing proper posture will reduce issues in all parts of the body, from head to toe.

The Green, Yellow, Red Zones

Too often people hurt their shoulder because they're not paying attention to how they're using it. If you've had a shoulder injury before, you should be particularly careful. One movement that commonly triggers a shoulder problem is simply reaching too far behind your "safe" zone. By staying mindful of the green, yellow, red zone concept, you can prevent further shoulder issues. The zones relate to three kinds of shoulder/arm movements: opening your arms (abduction), lifting your arms forward (flexion), and taking your arms backward (extension). Note that each arm/shoulder may have a different comfort zone and that changing hand position (e.g., turning your palms up, facing them inward) can affect mobility in one or both shoulders.

Most people can perform movements in the green zone. The green zone places the least amount of stress on your shoulder, and should be suffi-cient when doing any activity, including exercise and rehabil-itation. When your elbow/hand is in the yellow zone, there is moderate stress on your shoulder; caution should be used in this zone. When you reach into the red zone, the shoulder is under the most stress, making it unstable and vulnerable to injury. Try to avoid motions in the red zone when possible, especially if you have an injured shoulder.

To determine your zones when abducting your arms, start by standing with your back against a wall.

1. Raise your arms in front of you at shoulder height with your palms facing each other. Now spread them to just where you can't see your hands anymore. Does this hurt? If not, this is your *green zone*—you can perform most activities in this zone and not hurt yourself.

2. Now spread your hands back to the wall. Does this hurt? This is the *yellow zone*—this is where some people dis-play tightness. Whether or not you feel tightness, you should still be careful in this zone.

3. The *red zone* is behind you, such as when you reach into the back seat of the car without turning your body.

To determine your zones when moving your arms forward

(*shoulder flexion*), start by standing with your arms alongside your body.

1. Raise your arms forward to shoulder height with your palms facing each other. This area should move freely and is your *green zone*.

2. As you raise your arms above shoulder height, you may feel some restriction. This is your *yellow zone*.

3. Anything above and beyond your head is the *red zone*.

To determine your zones when moving your arms backward (shoulder extension), start by standing with your arms alongside your body.

1. Slowly move your arms straight back 3–4 inches. This should feel relatively comfortable and is your *green zone*.

2. The difference between the *yellow and red zones* is very small, so be careful any time you move your arm back and up (to scratch your upper back, for instance).

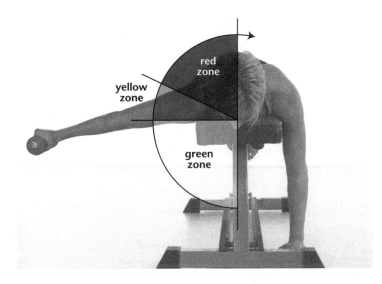

Shoulder abduction zones

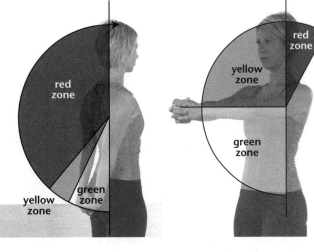

Shoulder extension zones   *Shoulder flexion zones*

Do's and Don'ts

Following these Do's and Don'ts can dramatically reduce shoulder injury:

Do

• Separate and lighten loads.
• Lift and carry loads close to your body.
• Take frequent breaks from any repetitive activity.

• Sleep on your back or your unaffected shoulder with a pillow between your arm and body. Watch that your shoulder stays in line with your body. You might also rest your affected arm on top of a pillow.
• Wear a fanny pack or sling your bag's strap across your

body and unaffected shoulder or tuck the load between your body and elbow.
• When performing activities that are shoulder intensive, such as sweeping or vacuuming, move your whole body by moving your feet and keep your arm tucked in close to your side. Take

small steps and keep your back straight.

- Use inexpensive "reachers" or grabber devices to protect your shoulder.
- Practice good posture.
- Rearrange your work station.
- Alternate the arm you use to carry your briefcase or purse.
- Pay close attention to how your head and upper back are positioned while at work and during activities of daily living.
- Make sure you're not placing too much load in your arms when you're sitting at your desk or work station.

Don't

- Don't slump and let your shoulder round forward.
- Don't work with your arms overhead for prolonged periods.
- Don't lift excessively heavy loads.
- Don't allow your hands to be out of your sight when your arms are out to the side.
- Don't reach far in front or in back of you to pick something up.
- Don't work for more than 15–20 minutes without a rest break for your shoulder.
- Don't sleep on your affected shoulder.

- Don't sling the strap of your purse or other load over your affected shoulder.
- Don't prop yourself up on your affected arm while reading or watching TV.
- Don't rest your affected arm on the car-door window ledge.
- Don't carry bags or pocketbooks on your shoulders.
- Don't overdo it in activities in which you normally don't participate. Train to play.

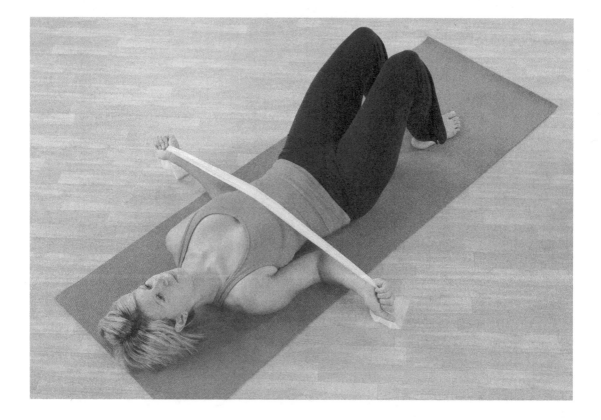

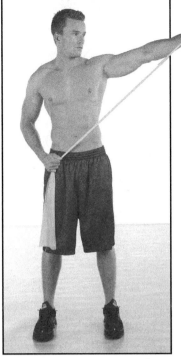

controversial exercises

Everyone knows that physical activity and exercise is good for the human body. Unfortunately, in our zest to get fit, we often hurt ourselves because we're using outdated principles or are driven by faulty assumptions. The fitness industry has evolved, but some exercises have been around so long that it seems irreverent to question their efficacy.

Many of us are bombarded with glitzy infomercials and celebrity endorsements that convey erroneous exercise facts. Successful coaches who have produced winning teams have also passed down some faulty myths. Often, training methods get adopted and later institutionalized based on anecdotal information rather than science.

Most of the controversial exercises discussed here will not kill you today or even really hurt you if done once or twice. The problem is cumula-tive and manifests itself over time. The human body is resilient, but if it's constantly misused and abused, the nega-tive effects of improper exercise will show up in later years.

One expert stated that at least 90 percent of exercise programs include some exer-cises that are as detrimental as they are valuable. The key when determining if an exer-cise is correct is whether or not it passes the benefits-to-risk ratio: Is this exercise doing more harm than good, and is there a safer, more effective way to get the desired results? A simple example that comes to mind is the traditional sit-up versus curl-up, or full squat versus lunge.

When you participate in a fitness routine, ask yourself the following questions:

- Why am I doing this exercise?
- What are the benefits of this exercise?
- What are the risks of this exercise?
- How do I feel while doing this exercise?

SHOULDER JOINT CONSIDERATIONS

According to orthopedic doctors, shoulder impingement is increasingly becoming a concern for exercisers. All movements involving the shoulder region need to be controlled, and the hands should be supinated (palms up) if raising the arms above shoulder height as this allows more space in the joint. Using hand weights with the arms fully extended can aggravate shoulder problems and may cause elbow problems as well. Relax the shoulders and retract the shoulder blades when performing arm exercises (there is a tendency to shrug the shoulders up near the ears when exercising the arms).

- How do I feel after doing this exercise?
- Could I receive the same benefits doing a different exercise?

If the answers to these questions are negative, look for another exercise routine. If your trainer fails to be mindful of the considerations above, find a different trainer. Similarly, if you come across a trainer who prescribes to outdated concepts (such as those noted below) or, better yet, says "No pain, no gain," RUN! Today, we maintain that the "no pain, no gain" concept is insane. You know how your body feels—listen to it and heed what it says.

Do not become complacent about exercise, especially if you've suffered an injury. It's critical for you to be mindful of proper body mechanics when working out and to associate with your body while working out. This involves paying attention to what you're doing and how the exercise affects your body. One thought to consider is not playing music while exercising because it's easy to forget about your form. Once the move is in your muscle memory, you can use music, but still focus on form. Remember: Only perfect practice makes perfect! Think PP, which stands for Perfect Posture. The key to injury prevention is to exercise smart, not hard. Any exercise that has made it into your routine should give maximum return on your investment.

You should be equally mindful when selecting an activity, an exercise or a piece of equipment. Ask yourself the following:

- Is it safe?
- Does the activity work the targeted muscle?
- Do the benefits outweigh the risks?
- Is the activity biomechanically correct?
- Does the exercise relate to the other exercises?

- How does it feel?
- Is it harming a joint?
- Does it take too much time to do?
- Does it accomplish what I want it to?

Any exercise done incorrectly can cause problems, but some common exercises are riskier than others. The following 13 exercises fail the "benefits to risk" index:

1. **Lat Pulls** when the bar is pulled down behind the neck or done too quickly and pulled down far below chin level.

2. **Military Presses** done behind the head/neck.

3. **Dumbbell Flys and Reverse Flys** done with the arms extremely wide (i.e., in the yellow and red zones).

4. **Bench Presses** with barbell or dumbbells held too wide or with the elbows dipping too far below or behind the bench. *Placing the hands in a more neutral grip puts less strain on the shoulder.*

5. **Lateral Raises and Frontal Raises** done too quickly or lifted higher than shoulder height.

6. **Upright Rows** when the bar is pulled too high.

7. **Shrugs** when done with improper grip width (too wide or too narrow) or when shoulders roll forward and drop quickly. *Shrugs when performed*

with a comfortable weight are OK.

8. **Bicep curls** done on a straight barbell. Instead, use a neutral grip. *Dumbbells would be a better choice when doing bicep curls.*

9. **Triceps** curls done with machines or performed with awkward positioning (e.g., French curls).

10. **Wide-grip pull-ups and pull-ups done behind the head.**

11. **Water exercise equipment or movements that replicate contraindicated weight exercises.** While water exercise is generally excellent and low impact, poor biomechanics and classes taught by ill-trained instructors can hurt you. In the water, the 3 S's determine resistance: *size* of the object, *speed* of the movement and *shape* of the object.

12. **Push-ups** when done too wide or done in a manner that strains your shoulder. *Push-ups done with hands in a neutral position are best.*

13. **Bar dips** done too low or too quickly.

Stay alert to the variables discussed here and you'll avoid a cervical neck, upper back or shoulder problem.

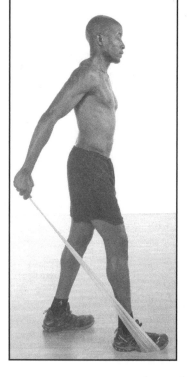

designing a shoulder routine

If you've read this book from the beginning, you'll have learned all about the shoulder's amazing mobility as well as its areas of vulnerability. The range of activities that could negatively affect the shoulder might even be discouraging to you.

However, rather than give up on swimming, playing tennis, or even painting your kitchen, you can continue doing what you enjoy by conditioning your body and maintaining a high level of fitness. Giving your shoulder a simple daily dose of TLC will provide a big return on investment.

Part 3 features a number of exercises designed to help you recover from an injury or maintain a healthy shoulder. Every effort was made to include only movements and

exercises recognized by shoulder experts and therapists. If you're in the early stages of your rehabilitation, you should follow your medical professional's recommendations to the letter for the best results. The exercises they prescribe may or may not be in this book, and that's fine. If you've fully recovered and have been discharged by your doctor, go ahead and select the exercises that appeal to you, changing them up periodically.

The advantage of having this book is that you can take it

with you to your therapist and ask her/him to highlight the exercises they'd like you to do and the ones you should avoid. It's important to remember that there is no perfect exercise for everyone, nor is there a perfect training routine. In functional fitness, everything should be adapted and individualized for your specific needs. This book can be a living document that will allow you to monitor, add and delete exercises as are appropriate.

The exercises you choose should be specific, purposeful

and goal oriented, with each movement contained within the program leading to greater independence and normalized function. Functional shoulder exercises should follow this progression:

- Large muscles to small muscles
- Simple movements to complex motions
- Static movements to dynamic motions
- Slow movements to fast motions
- Movements in a single plane to movements in multiple planes
- Low-force activities to high-force activities
- Dual-arm movements to single-arm motions
- Stable-surface drills to stability challengers

If you're in recovery mode, trial and error is the best approach. Start slowly and include some basic active exercises and stretches as well as a few corrective exercises. If you notice an increase in your symptoms, stop immediately and consult your health advisor.

If you don't have an existing shoulder issue, follow this basic protocol:

Stretches
- Beginners: Hold each stretch 10–15 seconds.

EXERCISE SAFETY TIPS

Early intervention to identify a problem keeps small problems small.

- Maintain a proper balance between training and proper rest.
- Balance your volume of training with intensity of training.
- Know your range of motion. Each of us has a unique range of motion of the shoulder—learn your safe range. One person's range may be another person's pain.
- Learn which exercises are high-risk exercises as they pertain to your shoulder.
- Always perform your exercises with proper execution.
- Learn various methods to cross-train to prevent overuse syndrome. Don't overtrain the same muscles in the same manner day in and day out (e.g., swimming for yards and yards every day).

- Always include exercises to train the small supporting muscles of your shoulder. Most of us focus on the "show" muscles and forget the importance of these smaller muscles.
- Understand the possible dangers of too many speed movements in your activity.
- Train smart, NOT heavy. Too much weight combined with poor execution equals injury!
- Understand how to mix reps and sets for maximum gain and minimum risk.
- Learn how to prepare for activity, whether it's pre-season conditioning or pre-game joint readiness.
- Learn how to adapt your training by including concepts of plyometrics, periodization, and open-kinetic- vs. closed-kinetic-chain moves.

- Advanced: Hold each stretch up to 1 minute.

Active Exercises
- Beginners: Start with 5 repetitions (reps).
- Advanced: Work up to 15 reps, then move on to another pain-free exercise.

As always, remember to warm up first and aim for quality motions over quantity. Before advancing to the next level, you should be able to correctly perform the skill's previous level. Advancing too quickly just because you're bored increases your risks for

a possible re-injury. Therapeutic exercises are not about increasing the load or length of stretch time each time—in this case, more is not better.

Whether or not you're nursing an existing injury, if you experience any increase in pain or symptoms, such as numbness or tingling, do not continue with any exercise from this book and consult your doctor. Your doctor's advice supersedes the information in this book because of his or her familiarity with your unique situation.

Sample Conditioning Programs

This section features shoulder programs for several sports and occupations. It also includes a program for general overall conditioning. Assuming you are pain free, locate the program that applies to you and perform it daily; a cross-training approach in which you stretch daily and do the conditioning exercises 2–3 times a week might also work well. Prior to doing any exercise, remember to warm up the joint area. A warm-up is not the same as stretching—a warm-up is simply any activity that increases muscle temperature so the joint is more limber. Tight muscles, ligaments and tendon are more inclined to be injured.

Determining how long to hold a stretch or how many reps to do to is truly an individual decision. There is no magic formula that will work for everyone. Each person will respond differently, and the old adage "pain will be your guide" has never been more true than with shoulder treat-ment. Avoid overdoing it; more is not always better. The bottom line is your shoulder will tell you how high to reach, how far to stretch, and how long to hold a stretch.

However, if you don't have an existing shoulder issue, you can follow the basic protocol noted on page 41. Some of the programs will suggest strengthening exercises that utilize a band or dumbbell. If you have one but not the other, feel free to do the exercise with the prop you have on hand.

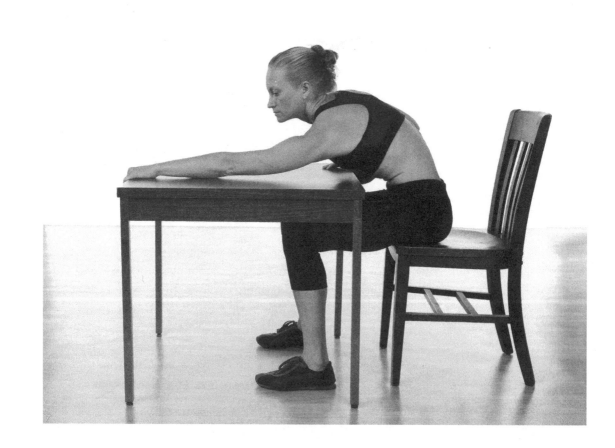

general conditioning

This program is designed to provide overall wellness to the shoulder complex. You won't build giant muscles or extreme flexibility doing these exercises; you'll simply keep your shoulders in good working order and prevent injuries from occurring. This program can be easily integrated into your usual exercise routine.

These exercises should be done after a thermal warm-up or after your workout.

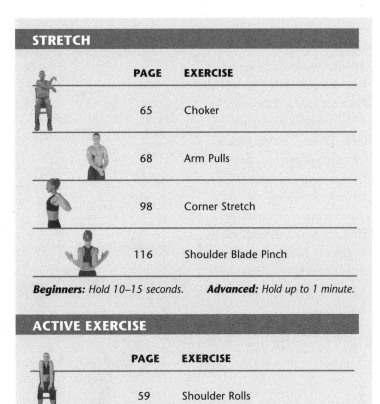

STRETCH

	PAGE	EXERCISE
	65	Choker
	68	Arm Pulls
	98	Corner Stretch
	116	Shoulder Blade Pinch

Beginners: *Hold 10–15 seconds.*　　**Advanced:** *Hold up to 1 minute.*

ACTIVE EXERCISE

	PAGE	EXERCISE
	59	Shoulder Rolls
	60	Elbow Touches
	130	Serving Tray
	131	Internal Rotation with Band

Beginners: *Start with 5 reps.*　　**Advanced:** *Work up to 15 reps.*

baseball/softball

Rotator cuff injuries and shoulder impingement concerns are the most common shoulder problems seen in throwing sports. Baseball pitchers have a higher incidence of shoulder problems than softball pitchers due to the mechanics of the pitch. However, infielders who do a great deal of repetitive infield work are at risk in both sports. To prevent an injury, perform *pre*-pre-season conditioning to prepare your body for hours of throwing.

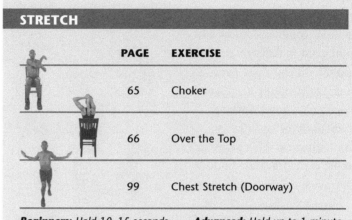

STRETCH

	PAGE	EXERCISE
	65	Choker
	66	Over the Top
	99	Chest Stretch (Doorway)

Beginners: Hold 10–15 seconds.   **Advanced:** Hold up to 1 minute.

ACTIVE EXERCISE

	PAGE	EXERCISE
	55	Arm Swings (Forward & Backward)
	125	Frontal Raises
	126	Lateral Raises
	128	T's with Band
	131	Internal Rotation with Band
	132	External Rotation with Band
	140	Dumbbell Shoulder Extension
	141	Dumbbell Soup Can Pours

Beginners: Start with 5 reps.   **Advanced:** Work up to 15 reps.

basketball

Although lower-body injuries are more common in basketball players, shoulder issues can still pop up when players aren't paying attention. Shooting too many baskets over a short period of time, in particular, may result in rotator cuff tendinitis.

STRETCH

PAGE	EXERCISE
65	Choker
66	Over the Top
99	Chest Stretch (Doorway)

Beginners: Hold 10–15 seconds. **Advanced:** Hold up to 1 minute.

ACTIVE EXERCISE

PAGE	EXERCISE
55	Arm Swings (Forward & Backward)
125	Frontal Raises
126	Lateral Raises
142	Reverse Fly
131	Internal Rotation with Band
132	External Rotation with Band
140	Dumbbell Shoulder Extension
141	Dumbbell Soup Can Pours

Beginners: Start with 5 reps. **Advanced:** Work up to 15 reps.

football

Shoulder dislocations are common in football. Pre-season conditioning should consist of strengthening the shoulder complex to provide as much stability and support as possible to the joint area.

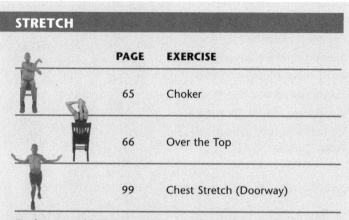

STRETCH

	PAGE	EXERCISE
	65	Choker
	66	Over the Top
	99	Chest Stretch (Doorway)

Beginners: *Hold 10–15 seconds.*   **Advanced:** *Hold up to 1 minute.*

ACTIVE EXERCISE

	PAGE	EXERCISE
	55	Arm Swings (Forward & Backward)
	139	Dumbbell Frontal Raises
	126	Lateral Raises
	142	Reverse Fly
	131	Internal Rotation with Band
	132	External Rotation with Band

Beginners: *Start with 5 reps.*   **Advanced:** *Work up to 15 reps.*

golf

Golf might look like a gentle enough sport, but when played often and/or without proper technique, it can lead to injury from overuse or misuse. Shoulder issues appear less frequently than back, elbow, hand and wrist problems, but plenty of golfers experience rotator cuff impingement. The following should be done prior to playing golf and in between holes.

STRETCH

	PAGE	EXERCISE
	91	Reverse Lift
	63	Picture Frame
	107	Isometric Shoulder Blade Squeeze
	114	Upper Back Stretch

Beginners: Hold 10–15 seconds.   **Advanced:** Hold up to 1 minute.

ACTIVE EXERCISE

	PAGE	EXERCISE
	56	Arm Swings (Across Body)
	58	Shoulder Box
	70	Elbow Touches (Supine)
	72	Straight-Arm Stretch
	85	Shoulder Slaps
	86	I's, Y's & T's on Roller

Beginners: Start with 5 reps.   **Advanced:** Work up to 15 reps.

hockey

The majority of hockey injuries result from direct trauma, whether through falls or player contact. Knee, hand and wrist injuries are the most common, but players are also subject to shoulder separations/dislocations. The best prevention for this is to strengthen the shoulder muscles as well as maintain flexibility.

STRETCH

	PAGE	EXERCISE
	65	Choker
	66	Over the Top
	99	Chest Stretch (Doorway)

Beginners: Hold 10–15 seconds.   **Advanced:** Hold up to 1 minute.

ACTIVE EXERCISE

	PAGE	EXERCISE
	58	Shoulder Box
	60	Elbow Touches
	139	Dumbbell Frontal Raises
	142	Reverse Fly

Beginners: Start with 5 reps.   **Advanced:** Work up to 15 reps.

swimming

Any sport that requires repetitive overhead motions has a high risk of injury. In swimming, the freestyle/crawl, backstroke and butterfly present the most risk. Strokes done with an underwater recovery, such as the breaststroke, are easier on the shoulder.

Consider doing underwater recovery strokes during rehab, and focus on techniques, kicks and quality workouts rather than high-volume workouts.

STRETCH

	PAGE	EXERCISE
	65	Choker
	66	Over the Top
	99	Chest Stretch (Doorway)
	67	Internal Rotation Stretch
	122	The Zipper

Beginners: Hold 10–15 seconds.   **Advanced:** Hold up to 1 minute.

ACTIVE EXERCISE

	PAGE	EXERCISE
	58	Shoulder Box
	60	Elbow Touches
	127	Shoulder Extension
	132	External Rotation with Band

Beginners: Start with 5 reps.   **Advanced:** Work up to 15 reps.

tennis

Tennis requires flexibility and power. Tennis serves count on the shoulder joint to perform at high speeds and at extreme ranges of motion. This combination sets the stage for bursitis and rotator cuff injuries. The backhand can also place the shoulder joint in awkward angles.

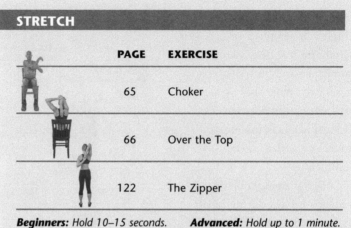

STRETCH

	PAGE	EXERCISE
	65	Choker
	66	Over the Top
	122	The Zipper

Beginners: *Hold 10–15 seconds.*   **Advanced:** *Hold up to 1 minute.*

ACTIVE EXERCISE

	PAGE	EXERCISE
	56	Arm Swings (Across Body)
	112	Soup Can Pours
	130	Serving Tray
	127	Shoulder Extension
	129	Sword Fighter
	132	External Rotation with Band

Beginners: *Start with 5 reps.*   **Advanced:** *Work up to 15 reps.*

volleyball

Volleyball players who serve and spike are at greater risk of injury than those who set the ball. Also, due to the nature of the sport, players are constantly diving for the ball, which presents opportunities for shoulder dislocation.

STRETCH

	PAGE	EXERCISE
	65	Choker
	66	Over the Top

Beginners: Hold 10–15 seconds.　　　　**Advanced:** Hold up to 1 minute.

ACTIVE EXERCISE

	PAGE	EXERCISE
	128	T's with Band
	137	Y's with Band
	129	Sword Fighter
	76	Crossing Guard
	141	Dumbbell Soup Can Pours

Beginners: Start with 5 reps.　　　　**Advanced:** Work up to 15 reps.

wrestling

Wrestling exposes players to major impact that can result in dislocations. Additionally, wrestlers' arms are commonly placed or forced in unnatural positions that overstretch the shoulder joint. Wrestlers need adequate strength and power along with flexibility in order to not get injured when they're stretched and pulled like Gumby, so make sure they do these exercises when they're not hefting heavy plates of lead.

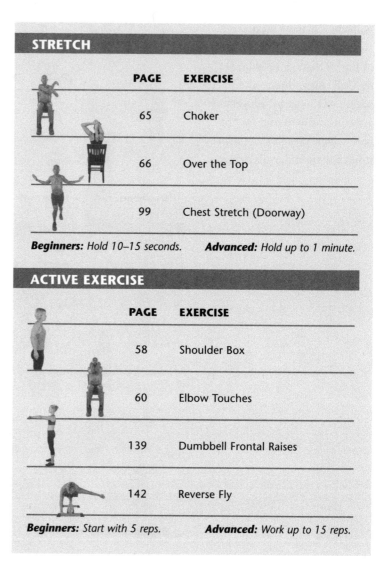

STRETCH

	PAGE	EXERCISE
	65	Choker
	66	Over the Top
	99	Chest Stretch (Doorway)

Beginners: Hold 10–15 seconds.   **Advanced:** Hold up to 1 minute.

ACTIVE EXERCISE

	PAGE	EXERCISE
	58	Shoulder Box
	60	Elbow Touches
	139	Dumbbell Frontal Raises
	142	Reverse Fly

Beginners: Start with 5 reps.   **Advanced:** Work up to 15 reps.

construction job

In construction, a worker's body is oftentimes also his tool. Workers who perform a lot of overhead work are at an increased risk for shoulder problems so they should take special care to do these exercises when they're not on the job.

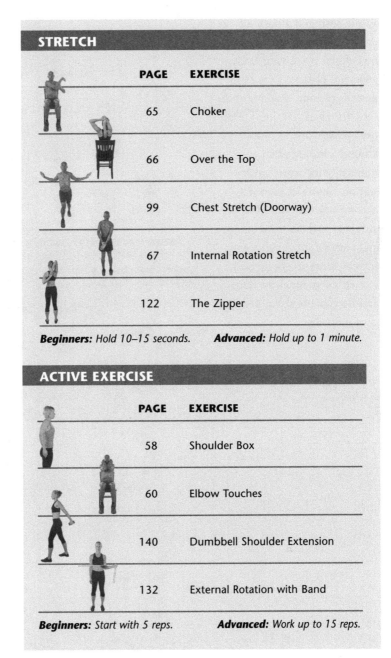

STRETCH

	PAGE	EXERCISE
	65	Choker
	66	Over the Top
	99	Chest Stretch (Doorway)
	67	Internal Rotation Stretch
	122	The Zipper

Beginners: *Hold 10–15 seconds.*   ***Advanced:*** *Hold up to 1 minute.*

ACTIVE EXERCISE

	PAGE	EXERCISE
	58	Shoulder Box
	60	Elbow Touches
	140	Dumbbell Shoulder Extension
	132	External Rotation with Band

Beginners: *Start with 5 reps.*   ***Advanced:*** *Work up to 15 reps.*

office/desk job

While sitting at a desk all day isn't particularly strenuous, it can place your body in awkward positions for long periods of time. Pay attention to whether or not you hunch over paperwork or move around a mouse at an ergonomically incorrect work station. Shoulder pain may accompany common desk-job ailments such as neck strain and carpal tunnel syndrome, so remember to get up and stretch a few times an hour and be vigilant about keeping good posture.

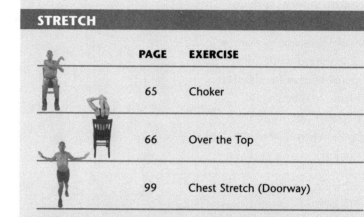

STRETCH

	PAGE	EXERCISE
	65	Choker
	66	Over the Top
	99	Chest Stretch (Doorway)

Beginners: Hold 10–15 seconds.   *Advanced:* Hold up to 1 minute.

ACTIVE EXERCISE

	PAGE	EXERCISE
	55	Arm Swings (Forward & Backward)
	125	Frontal Raises
	126	Lateral Raises
	128	T's with Band
	131	Internal Rotation with Band
	132	External Rotation with Band
	140	Dumbbell Shoulder Extension
	141	Dumbbell Soup Can Pours

Beginners: Start with 5 reps.   *Advanced:* Work up to 15 reps.

shoulder
conditioning
exercises

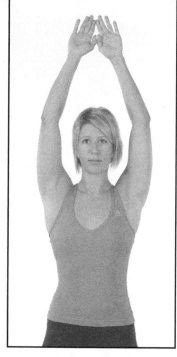

the exercises

The exercises in this chapter are grouped according to the position in which the exercise is performed, or its purpose. For instance, exercises that are done while standing are presented together. Generally, the exercises are listed in progression from easiest to most challenging. While the focus of each exercise is to restore function to your affected shoulder, it is advised that you perform the exercises bilaterally to prevent an injury to the other shoulder.

As you embark on the recovery process, you need to become your own personal trainer. The goal of a good trainer is to do NO harm. As a good trainer, you need to train smart—not hard. Avoid any activity that aggravates your shoulder. Pain is your body's way of informing you that something is going on internally. Never mask your pain with medications or lotions. To prevent a re-injury or unnecessary pain, execute motions with proper form.

The Two-Hour Rule

If your body hurts more than two hours post-workout, you did too much and need to rest until you can find a workout that is pain-free. If you suspect a re-injury, schedule a follow-up appointment with your doctor ASAP. Speak with your doctor/therapist about how and when you should heat and/or ice the affected area.

passive & gentle series

Prior to performing these motions, externally warm up the shoulder area, either by taking a warm shower or applying a moist heat pack. Consult your doctor first as to how you should warm up the joint. Use caution when applying heat to the area to avoid a burn.

arm swings (forward & backward)   *shoulder*

Goal: increase range of flexion and extension

STARTING POSITION: Place your unaffected arm on a table or other stable surface for support and lean over.

starting position

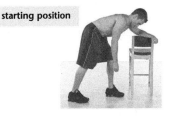

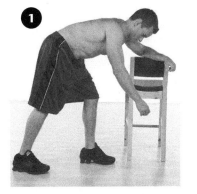

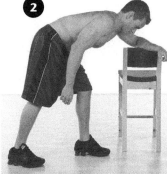

1–2 Gently swing your affected arm back and forth several times along the side of your body. Use your shoulder muscles, rather than your arm, to pull the arm down.

3 If you experience no pain, gradually increase the swings.

Switch sides and repeat.

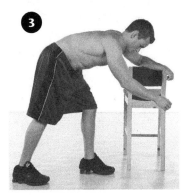

VARIATION: For additional traction, hold a dumbbell.

Goal: increase range of adduction and abduction

STARTING POSITION: Place your unaffected arm on a table or other stable surface for support and lean over.

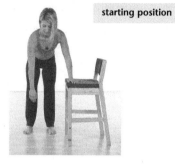

starting position

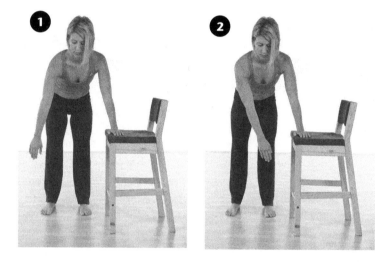

1–2 Gently swing your affected arm right and left several times across your body. Use your shoulder muscles, rather than your arm, to pull the arm down.

3 If you experience no pain, gradually increase the width of your swings.

Switch sides and repeat.

VARIATION: For additional traction, hold a dumbbell.

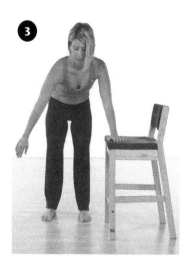

Goal: increase general range of motion

STARTING POSITION: Place your unaffected arm on a table or other stable surface for support and lean over.

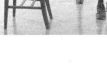
starting position

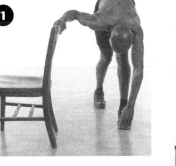

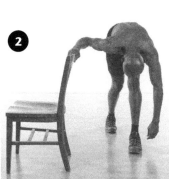

1–2 Gently swing your affected arm several times in a small, clockwise direction. Use your shoulder muscles, rather than your arm, to pull the arm down.

3–4 If you experience no pain, gradually increase circle size.

Gently swing your arm in a small, counterclockwise direction, then switch sides and repeat.

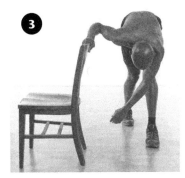

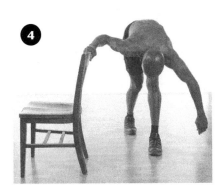

Goal: increase flexibility and prepare shoulder for sports play

STARTING POSITION: Stand tall with proper posture.

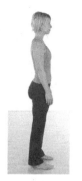

starting position

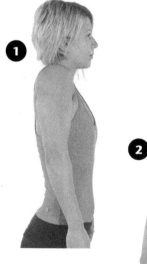

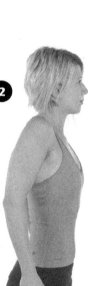

1 Inhaling deeply through your nose, slowly shrug your shoulders up to your ears.

2 Pull your shoulders back and squeeze the shoulder blades together and down.

3 Exhaling through your mouth, lower your shoulders and return to starting position.

Repeat as desired.

Goal: warm up the shoulder joint

STARTING POSITION: Sit with proper posture in a stable chair. Inhale slowly and deeply through your nose.

starting position

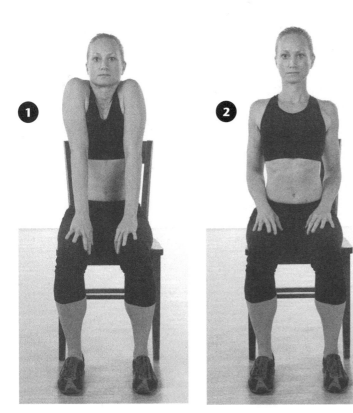

1 Roll your shoulders forward, attempting to touch your shoulders together.

2 Squeeze your shoulder blades together, moving your shoulders back and opening your chest.

Repeat as desired.

VARIATION: You can also perform the exercise while standing with proper posture.

Goal: warm up the shoulder joint

STARTING POSITION: Sit with proper posture in a stable chair. Place your left hand on your left shoulder and your right hand on your right shoulder.

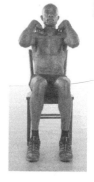

starting position

1 Slowly bring your elbows together in front of your body.

2 Bring your elbows out to the side while squeezing your shoulder blades together. Hold for a moment, focusing on opening up your chest. Return your elbows to starting position.

Repeat as desired.

VARIATION: Perform while standing with proper posture.

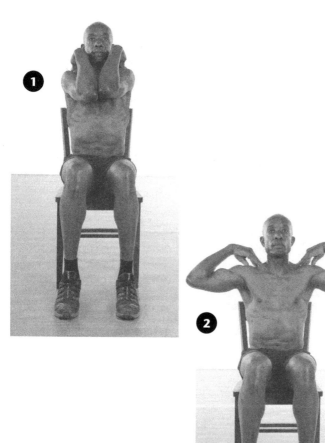

Goal: increase shoulder girdle flexibility

STARTING POSITION: Sit with proper posture in a stable chair. Clasp your hands behind your head.

starting position

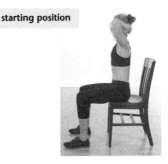

1 Slowly move your elbows backwards while bringing your shoulder blades together. Focus on opening up your chest and tightening your upper back muscles. Only go as far back as is comfortable and hold for a moment.

Return to starting position.

Repeat as desired.

VARIATION

A partner can help you increase the stretch by gently and slowly taking your elbows back. Use extreme caution when performing partner stretches.

apple pickers

deltoids

Goal: increase shoulder mobility

STARTING POSITION: Stand tall with proper posture and place your left hand on your left shoulder and your right hand on your right shoulder.

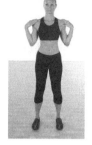
starting position

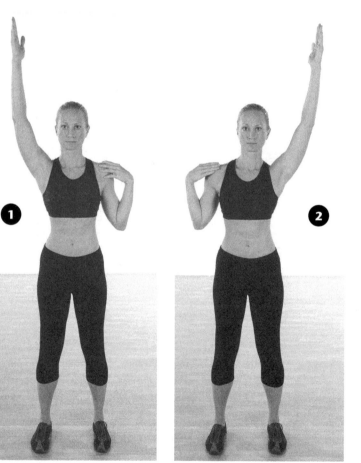

1 Move your right hand up to the ceiling.

2 Place your right hand back on your right shoulder and move your left hand up to the ceiling.

Continue alternating sides.

Goal: increase mobility

STARTING POSITION: Stand with proper posture. Place your right hand on your left elbow and your left hand on your right elbow.

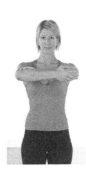

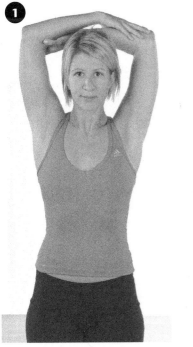

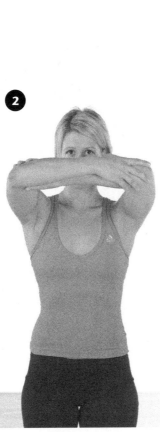

1 Slowly raise your arms overhead, lifting your arms no higher than your comfort level; make sure not to arch your back. Hold the position for a moment. You are now framing your face in a picture frame created by your arms— smile.

2 Return to starting position.

Repeat as desired.

VARIATION: This can also be performed while sitting with proper posture in a stable chair.

Goal: increase range of motion

STARTING POSITION: Sit with proper posture at a table and place your affected arm on the table.

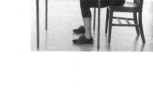

1 Slowly slide your arm forward across the table as if reaching towards the other side.

Switch sides and repeat.

Goal: increase range of motion

STARTING POSITION: Sit with proper posture in a stable chair.

starting position

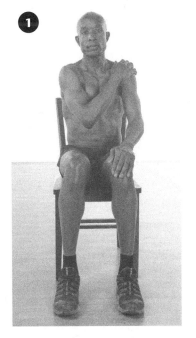

1 Place your right hand on your left shoulder.

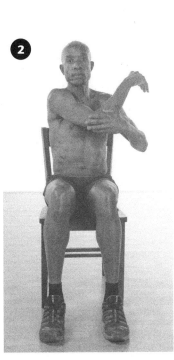

2 Place your left hand on your right elbow and gently press your right elbow toward your throat. Your elbow should be in line with your nose. Hold for a moment.

Switch sides and repeat.

VARIATION: Perform while standing with proper posture.

Goal: increase flexibility

STARTING POSITION: Sit with proper posture in a stable chair.

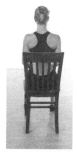

starting position

1 Reach your right hand up to the ceiling.

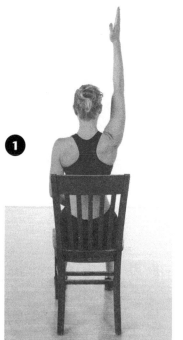

2 Bend your arm and let your forearm rest against the back of your head. Place your left hand on your right elbow and gently press your right arm down your back as far as feels comfortable. Hold for a moment.

Switch sides and repeat.

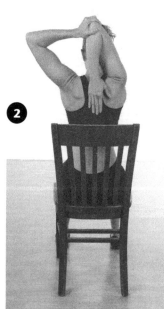

VARIATION: Perform while standing with proper posture.

Goal: increase range of internal rotation

STARTING POSITION: Stand tall with proper posture and place both arms behind your back. Grab your affected arm's wrist with the unaffected arm.

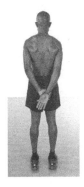

starting position

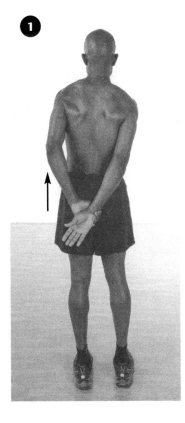

1 Gently push the affected arm up the spine. Do not force it!

68

passive & gentle series
arm pulls
joint space of the shoulder

Goal: provide gentle traction

STARTING POSITION: Stand tall with proper posture. Place a soft pad against your ribs, between your affected arm and torso. Place your affected arm in front of your body and grasp your affected wrist with your unaffected hand.

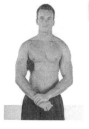

starting position

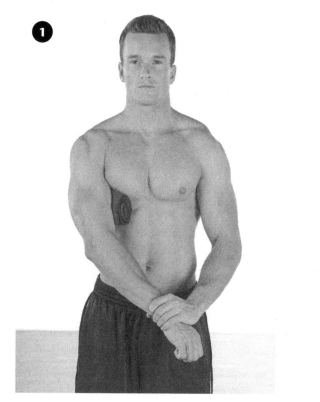

1 Gently pull your arm down and across your body. Hold for 5-10 seconds.

Repeat as desired.

VARIATION: You can also try the arm pull by taking the affected arm behind your back.

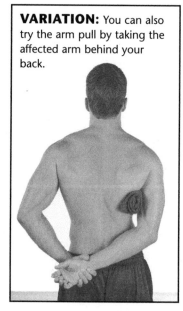

Goal: open up shoulder girdle

Note: This is a controversial exercise. Consult your doctor before attempting.

STARTING POSITION: Stand with your back against a solid table and place both palms on the edge of the table. If you feel discomfort, STOP!

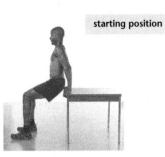

starting position

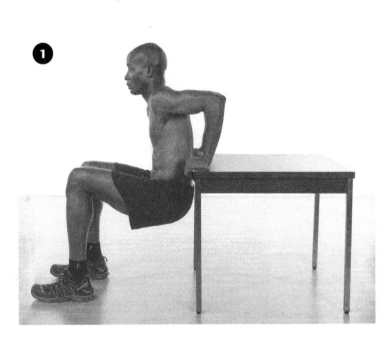

1 Bending your knees, slowly lower your buttocks towards the floor to enhance the stretch. Only go as far as feels comfortable—do not force it!

Return to starting position.

floor series

This series of exercises can be done on the floor or in your bed.

elbow touches (supine)

chest, upper back

Goal: increase range of shoulder motion, stretch chest muscles, strengthen upper back muscles

STARTING POSITION: Lie on your back, bend your knees and place your feet on the floor/bed. Clasp your hands behind your head.

starting position

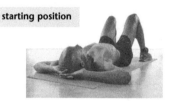

1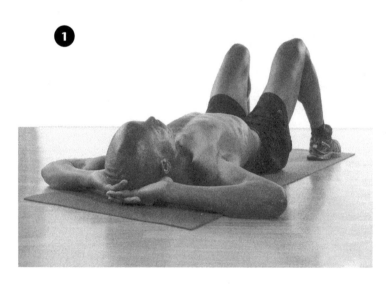

1 Gently press your elbows towards the floor or bed while squeezing your shoulder blades together. Stay within a comfortable pain zone; you'll feel a stretching sensation in the chest area. Hold for 2–5 seconds.

Goal: increase range of motion

STARTING POSITION: Lie on your back, bend your knees and place your feet on the floor/bed. Extend your affected arm up towards the ceiling, palm facing inward.

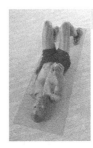

starting position

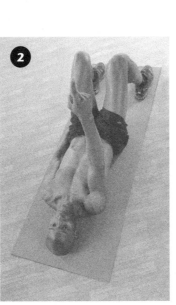

1–3 Slowly move your arm in small circles, as if you're drawing circles on the ceiling with your fingers. Keep your shoulder blades together.

Increase the size of the circle and then reverse directions.

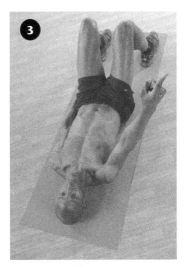

Goal: increase range of motion and flexibility of shoulder girdle

STARTING POSITION: Lie on your back, bend your knees and place your feet on the floor/bed. Extend your affected arm towards the ceiling with your thumb pointing back and palm facing inward. Try to keep your shoulder blades retracted together and your shoulders glued to the floor.

starting position

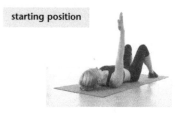

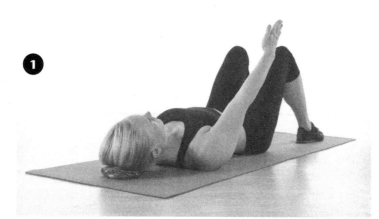

1–2 Keeping your arm straight the entire time, slowly move your pinky down next to your body, then slowly extend your arm back over your head, attempting to get your thumb comfortably close to the floor. Don't force the motion in either direction.

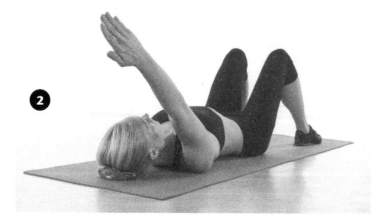

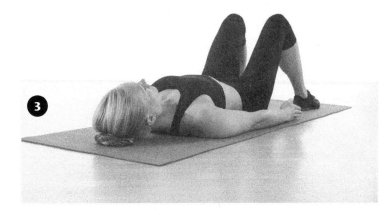

3 — 4 Repeat the movement, attempting to increase your range each time.

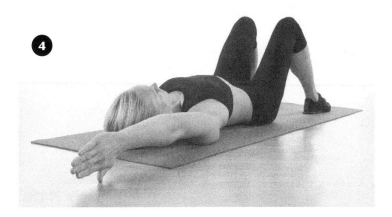

Goal: increase range of motion

STARTING POSITION: Lie on your back, bend your knees and place your feet on the floor or bed to keep your back in neutral position. Raise both arms towards the ceiling, palms facing inward.

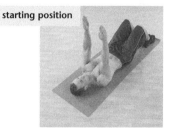

starting position

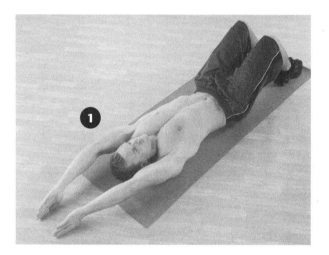

1 Keeping your back flat, slowly take both arms directly backwards, staying within your comfortable range of motion. From a top view, your arms will look like an "I" formation.

2 Return to starting position.

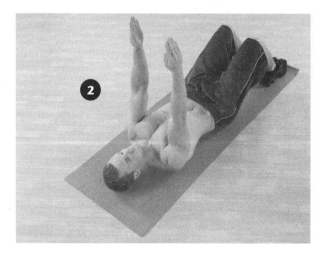

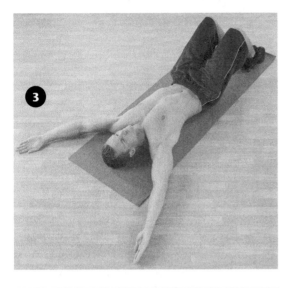

3 Now take both arms back and slightly out to the sides at a 45-degree angle, forming a "Y" shape.

4 Return to starting position.

5 Now slowly open both arms directly to the sides to form a "T" shape.

Return to starting position.

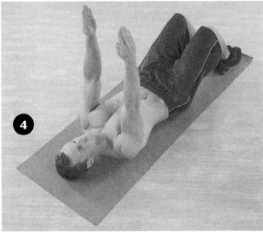

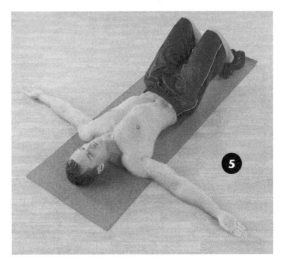

Goal: increase external rotation

STARTING POSITION: Lie on your back, bend your knees and place your feet on the floor/bed. Rest your elbows on the floor/bed. Bend your arms 90 degrees so that your forearms are perpendicular to your body and your fingers are pointing towards the ceiling, palms facing forward.

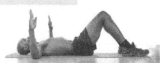
starting position

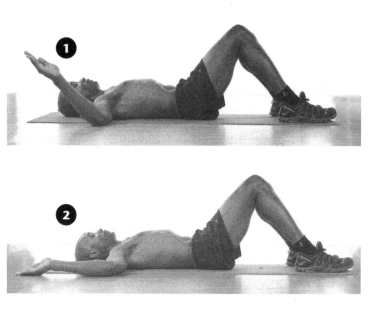

1–2 Slowly allow the backs of your hands to drop towards the floor. *Caution:* Most people are very tight in this region—stay within your comfort zone.

3 Slowly bring the palms of your hands forward to the floor.

Return to starting position.

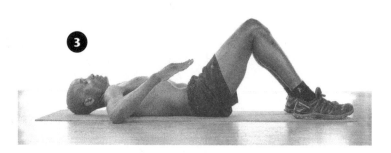

Goal: increase external rotation, strengthen rotator cuff

STARTING POSITION: Lie on your back, bend your knees and place your feet on the floor/bed. Rest your elbows on the floor. Bend your arms 90 degrees so that your forearms are perpendicular to your body and your fingers are pointing towards the ceiling, palms facing inward.

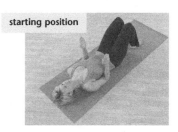

starting position

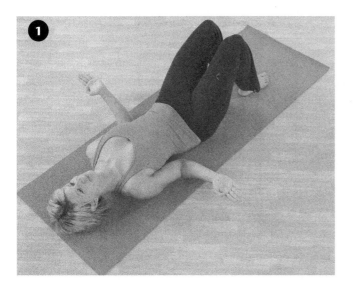

1 Slowly allow the backs of your hands to drop toward the floor. *Caution:* Most people are inflexible in this region. Don't force it—stay within your comfort zone.

Return to starting position.

VARIATION: For an additional challenge, hold the ends of a band in each hand.

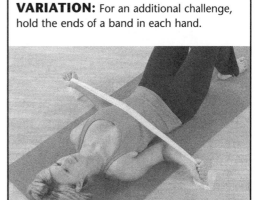

internal rotation (supine)
rotator cuff

Goal: increase internal rotation, strengthen rotator cuff muscles

STARTING POSITION: Lie on your back, bend your knees and place your feet on the floor/bed. Rest your elbows on the floor. Bend your arms 90 degrees so that your forearms are perpendicular to your body and your fingers point towards the ceiling, palms facing inward.

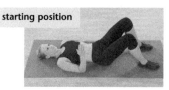
starting position

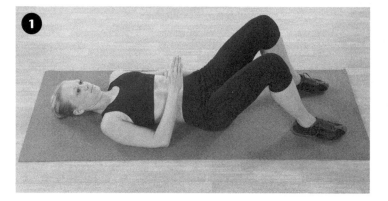

1 Keeping your elbows on the floor, slowly allow the palms of your hands to drop inward towards your belly button. Don't force it—be sure to stay within a comfortable zone.

Return to starting position.

Goal: increase internal rotation

STARTING POSITION: Lie on your affected side with your elbow against your torso and the back of your hand on the floor/bed. Bend your arm so that your forearm is perpendicular to your body. You may want to place a small rolled-up towel against your ribs.

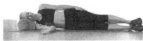

starting position

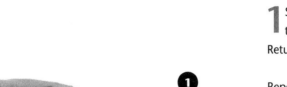

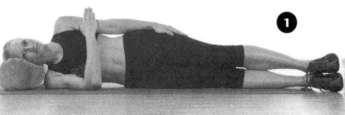

1 Slowly lift your fist up towards your belly. Return to starting position.

Repeat, then switch sides.

VARIATION: For an additional challenge, try holding a dumbbell.

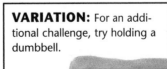

external rotation (side-lying) — *rotator cuff*

Goal: increase external rotation

STARTING POSITION: Lie on your unaffected side. Rest your affected elbow on your rib cage, with your arm bent in an L position; make a fist. Your palm will face the floor. You may want to place a small rolled-up towel between your torso and your elbow.

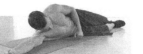

starting position

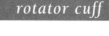

1 Slowly lift your fist up and back as high as possible. Don't force it or move rapidly.

Return to starting position.

Repeat, then switch sides.

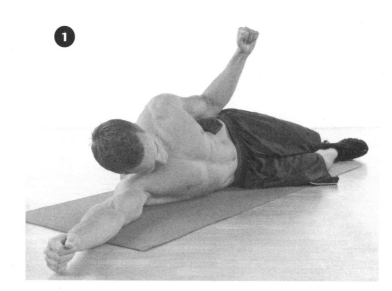

①

VARIATION: For an additional challenge, try holding a dumbbell.

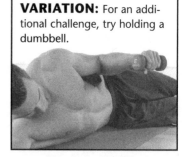

Goal: stabilize shoulder blades

STARTING POSITION: Assume a push-up position either on your knees or toes, keeping a nice line from the top of your head to your feet.

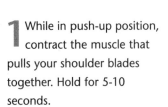

starting position

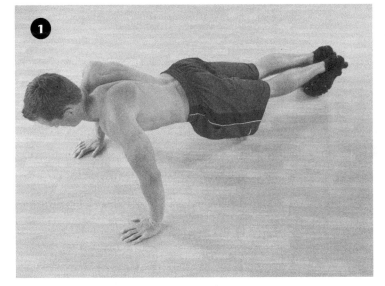

1

1 While in push-up position, contract the muscle that pulls your shoulder blades together. Hold for 5-10 seconds.

Release and relax.

VARIATION: To reduce the weight in your arms, try this from your knees or by leaning against a counter top.

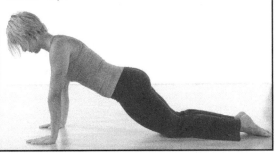

roller series

This section utilizes the foam roller, which provides an unstable surface that will challenge the stabilizer muscles of the body more than if you were to do the exercises without the prop. These exercises should only be done when you are symptom-free and desiring to challenge yourself.

First, you'll need to safely lie on a roller. Here's how you do it:

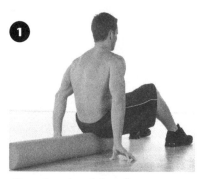

Sit on the edge of the roller.

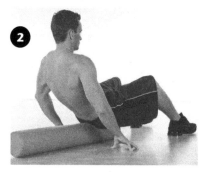

Slowly roll down your spine until your entire back is lying on the roller.

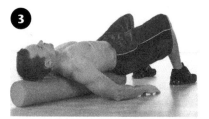

Your entire head should also be completely supported.

Goal: increase range of motion and stabilization of shoulder

STARTING POSITION: Lie on a foam roller, resting your head and the entire length of your back on it. Bend your knees and place your feet on the floor; place your arms on the floor alongside your body for balance. Breathe naturally and allow adequate time for your chest and shoulder region to relax and open up. For many people, this is an adequate stretch and it's OK to stop here without progressing to the following steps.

starting position

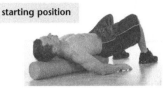

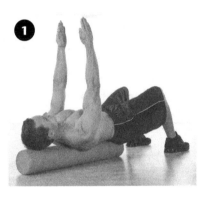

1 Once comfortable and stable, extend both arms up to the ceiling while maintaining balance on the roller; your palms should face each other. Be sure to stabilize your core the entire time by contracting your abs.

2 Allow one arm to move forward and the other backwards. Stay within your comfortable range of motion.

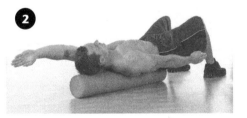

3 Reverse direction.

Release and relax.

Goal: open chest and shoulder girdle

STARTING POSITION: Lie on a foam roller, resting your head and the entire length of your back on it. Bend your knees and place your feet on the floor; place your arms on the floor alongside your body for balance. Breathe naturally and allow adequate time for your chest and shoulder area to relax and open up. For many people, this is an adequate enough stretch and it's OK to stop here without progressing to the following steps.

starting position

1 Once comfortable, place your hands under your head and slowly allow your elbows to "drop" towards the floor. You should not expect to touch the floor. Stop if this is uncomfortable. Hold the stretch while breathing naturally.

Release and relax.

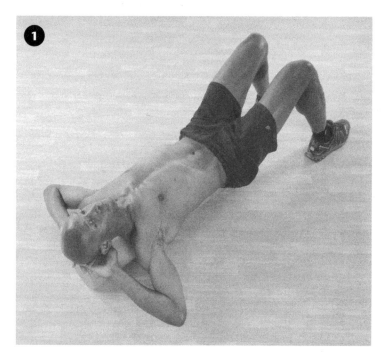

Goal: realign the shoulder girdle

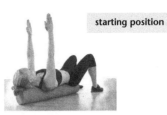

starting position

STARTING POSITION: Lie on a foam roller, resting your head and the entire length of your back on it. Bend your knees and place your feet on the floor; extend your arms up to the ceiling, palms facing each other.

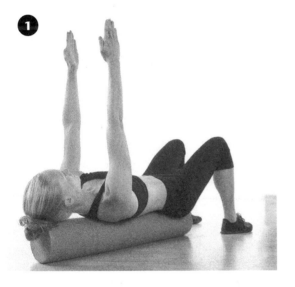

1 Reach your fingers up to the ceiling, allowing your shoulder blades to come off the roller.

2 Keeping your arms straight, completely relax your shoulder muscles, allowing your shoulder blades to "slap" back down on the roller.

Repeat as desired.

Goal: increase shoulder flexibility and stabilization

Caution: *This is an advanced exercise. Do not do this exercise until you have completed the I's, Y's and T's (page 74) on a solid surface.*

STARTING POSITION: Lie on a foam roller, resting your head and the entire length of your back on it. Bend your knees and place your feet on the floor; place your arms on the floor alongside your body for balance. Breathe naturally and allow adequate time for your chest and shoulder area to relax and open up. Focus on opening up the shoulder girdle and keeping your shoulders back. For many people, this is an adequate enough stretch and it's OK to stop here without progressing to the following steps.

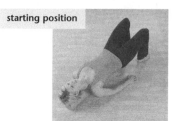

starting position

1 Once comfortable, extend both arms up towards the ceiling.

2 Now move both arms directly back and forth, making an "I," while focusing on shoulder blade stabilization.

3 Relax in starting position.

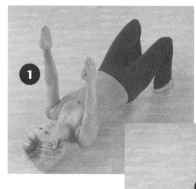

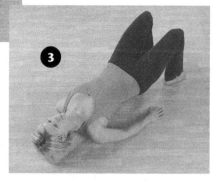

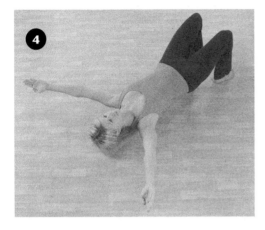

4 After completing the I's, take both arms slightly back and out to the sides at a 45-degree angle, forming a "Y" shape.

5 Relax in starting position.

6 After completing the Y's, slowly open both arms directly to the sides to form a "T" shape.

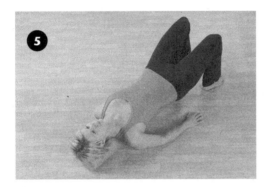

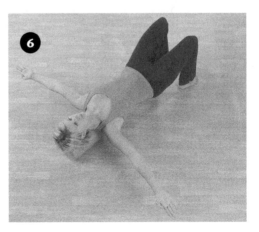

cane series

To assist your affected arm, this series of exercises uses a stick, cane or belt. The purpose of these exercises is to maintain or improve range of motion.

shoulder press (supine) — *shoulder, chest*

Goal: foster range of motion

STARTING POSITION: Lie on your back, bend your knees and place your feet on the floor. Grasp the stick or cane with each hand, shoulder-width apart, so that the stick is above your chest. Keep your elbows on the floor, close to your body.

starting position

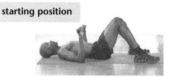

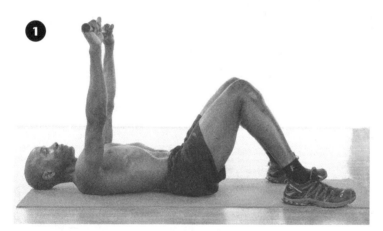

1 Press the stick up to the ceiling until both arms are fully extended.

Return to starting position.

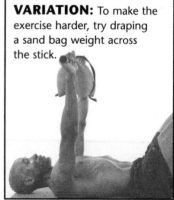

VARIATION: To make the exercise harder, try draping a sand bag weight across the stick.

Goal: foster range of motion

STARTING POSITION: Lie on your back, bend your knees and place your feet on the floor. Grasp the stick or cane with each hand, shoulder-width apart, so that the stick rests across your chest.

starting position

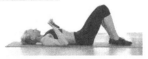

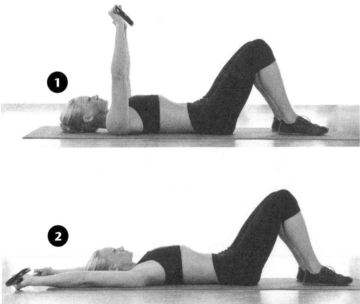

1 Press the stick up to the ceiling until both arms are fully extended.

2 Keeping your arms straight, slowly lower the stick behind your head and towards the floor. Do not force it!

3 Return to center.

VARIATION: To make the exercise harder, try draping a sand bag weight across the stick.

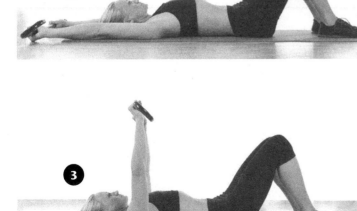

cane series
lateral drops

Goal: foster range of motion

STARTING POSITION: Lie on your back, bend your knees and place your feet on the floor. Grasp the stick or cane with each hand, shoulder-width apart, so that the stick rests across your chest.

starting position

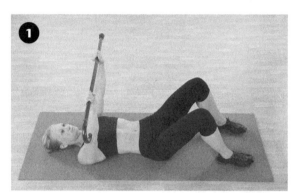

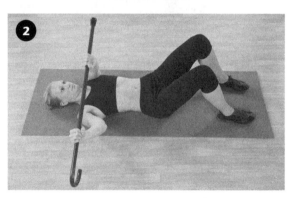

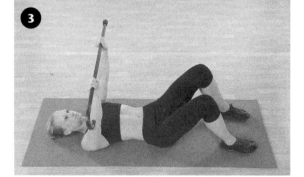

1 Press the stick up to the ceiling until both arms are fully extended.

2 Keeping your arms as straight as possible and your shoulder blades close to your spine, slowly lower the stick to the right side as far as you comfortably can. Try to keep both shoulders on the floor.

3 Return to center and "reset" your shoulder blades (pull your shoulder blades together to gently push your chest upwards).

Repeat on the other side.

Goal: increase range of motion

STARTING POSITION: Stand tall with proper posture. Grasp a strap, stick or cane behind your buttocks with your hands shoulder-width apart.

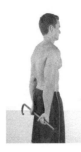

starting position

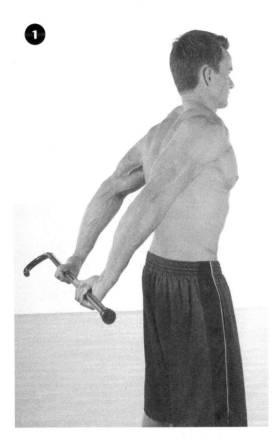

1 Keeping your arms straight, attempt to lift them away from your body. Focus on squeezing your shoulder blades together. Hold this position for as long as it's comfortable.

Return to starting position.

ADVANCED: Instead of using a device, interlock your hands behind your back and perform the movement.

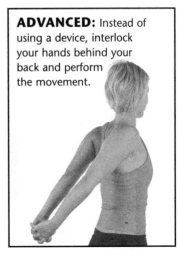

cane series
stick press

Goal: increase range of motion and improve shoulder strength

STARTING POSITION: Stand tall with proper posture. With both hands, hold the stick or cane against your chest at shoulder height, palms facing forward.

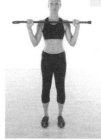

starting position

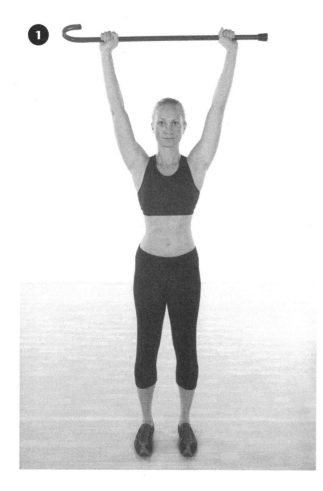

1 Press the stick up towards the ceiling as high as you comfortably can. Avoid arching your back to increase the height. If keeping your arms straight stresses your joints too much, you can press up with your arms angled.

Return to starting position.

VARIATION: This exercise can also be performed while seated and/or with a sand bag weight draped across the device.

Goal: increase internal range of motion

STARTING POSITION: Stand tall with proper posture and hold on to the cane or stick with both hands behind your buttocks.

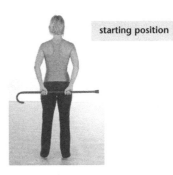

starting position

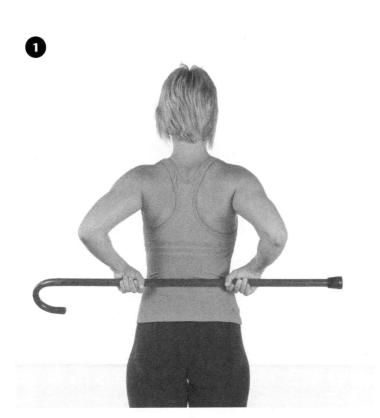

1

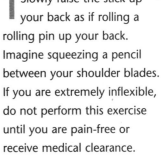

1 Slowly raise the stick up your back as if rolling a rolling pin up your back. Imagine squeezing a pencil between your shoulder blades. If you are extremely inflexible, do not perform this exercise until you are pain-free or receive medical clearance.

Return to starting position.

wall/door series

This series of exercises utilizes a door, doorframe, table or wall as a support prop to facilitate the activity.

finger walking (forward)   *shoulder*

Goal: increase flexion

STARTING POSITION: Face a wall and stand an arm's length away from it. Reach with the fingertips of your affected arm to touch the wall at shoulder height.

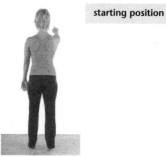

starting position

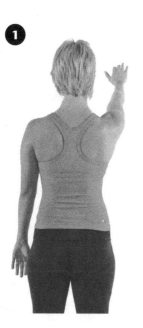

1

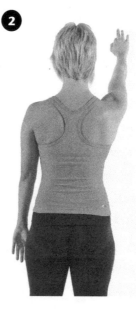

2

1–2 Slowly walk your fingers up the wall as high as you comfortably can. Do not arch your back or twist your body to gain height.

Return to starting position. Switch sides and repeat.

finger walking (side) *shoulder*

Goal: increase abduction

STARTING POSITION: Using your affected shoulder, stand sideways to a wall that is an arm's length away. Reach with your fingertips to touch the wall just below shoulder level.

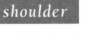
starting position

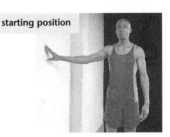

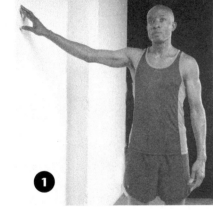

1–2 Slowly allow your fingers to walk up the wall as high as you comfortably can. Do not lean or elevate your shoulder to gain additional height.

Return to starting position. Switch sides and repeat.

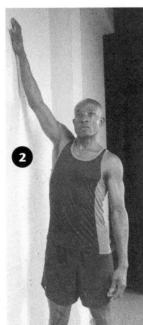

Goal: increase flexion/extension

STARTING POSITION: Using your affected shoulder, stand sideways to a wall that is an arm's length away. Stretch your affected arm straight up the wall (12 o'clock position).

starting position

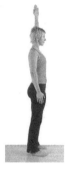

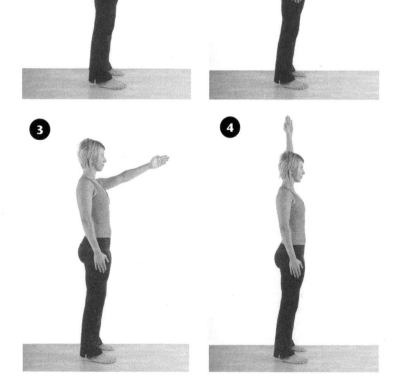

1 Slowly move your arm down the wall to the 3 o'clock position.

2 Return to 12 o'clock.

3 Slowly move to the 2 o'clock. Do not force it if you're inflexible!

4 Return to starting position.

Switch sides and repeat. Your arm will now point to the 9, 12 and 10 o'clock positions.

Goal: increase circumduction/rotation

STARTING POSITION: Face a wall and stand an arm's length away from it. Touch the wall with the index finger of your affected arm.

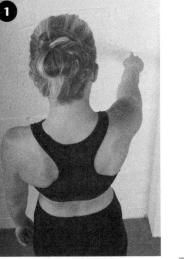

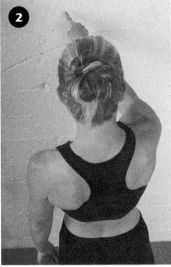

1–2 Slowly draw a small circle clockwise. If comfortable, make increasingly larger circles.

Reverse directions, making the circles progressively smaller. Switch sides and repeat.

wall/door series
corner stretch

chest, shoulder

Goal: increase chest and shoulder flexibility

STARTING POSITION: Start with your spine along the edge of a wall's corner. Focus on keeping your lower back and head against the corner. Breathe naturally.

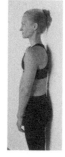

starting position

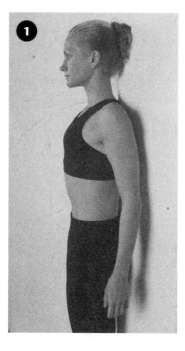

1 Slowly allow your shoulder blades to wrap around the corner with the goal of opening up the chest area. Hold for 5-10 seconds.

2 If possible, place your hands on your shoulders and gently enhance the stretch by pulling your elbows back with the muscles of your upper back. Hold for 5-10 seconds. If this is uncomfortable, do not force it.

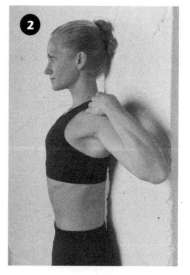

Goal: increase shoulder flexibility

STARTING POSITION: Stand in the middle of a doorframe. Place your hands on each side of the doorframe at a comfortable height.

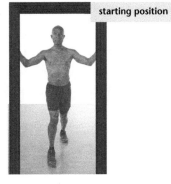

starting position

1 Slowly lean forward, allowing your body weight to stretch the front of your shoulders. Hold for 20–30 seconds.

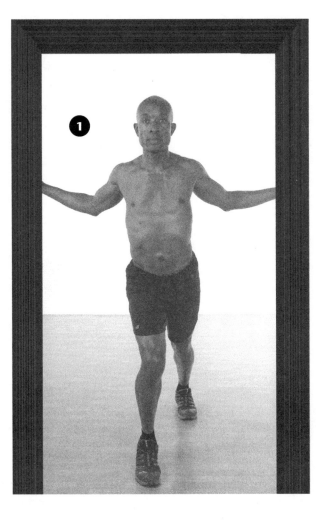

VARIATION: If a doorway is not available, ask a partner to grab your wrists and gently pull your arms behind you.

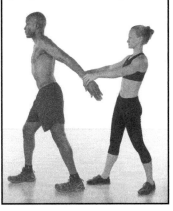

stick up

Goal: open up chest and shoulder region and tone functional shoulder muscle

STARTING POSITION: Stand with your back and head against the wall. Bend your arms 90 degrees, placing the backs of your hands on the wall. Hold for 3-5 seconds.

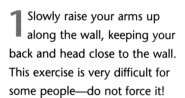

starting position

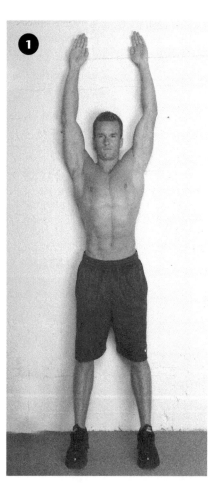

1 Slowly raise your arms up along the wall, keeping your back and head close to the wall. This exercise is very difficult for some people—do not force it!

elbow touches (against wall) — *pectorals*

Goal: increase shoulder girdle flexibility

STARTING POSITION: Stand with your back and head against the wall. Place your hands on your shoulders and point your elbows forward.

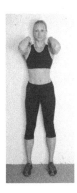

starting position

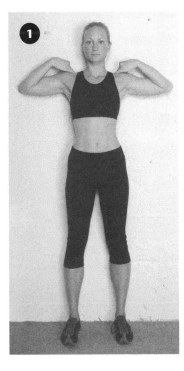

1 Carefully move your elbows towards the wall. Don't arch your back to increase your range. Touching the wall is not critical—the goal is to feel a gentle stretch in your chest and shoulders.

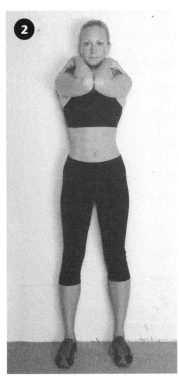

2 Slowly move your elbows back to center until you can touch them together.

Return to starting position.

double-hand press

Goal: increase strength in upper back

STARTING POSITION: Stand with your back and head against the wall and your arms along your sides. Place your palms on the wall.

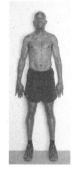

starting position

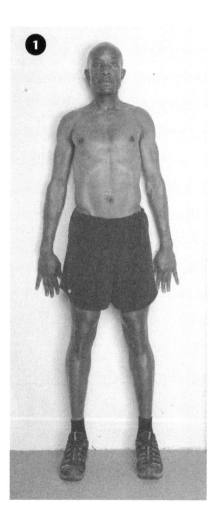

1 Gently press your hands against the wall, feeling the muscles between your shoulder blades contract. Do not hold your breath or arch your back.

Goal: passively stretch shoulder

STARTING POSITION: Stand against the edge of a wall and extend your affected arm along it. Feel the stretch through the shoulder area and relax and breathe freely.

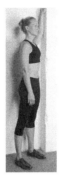

starting position

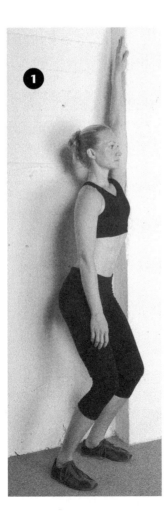

1 To enhance the stretch, slightly bend your knees to lower your body.

VARIATION: This can also be done against a doorframe.

Goal: increase external rotation strength

STARTING POSITION: Stand against a wall. Bend the elbow of your affected arm 90 degrees, keeping your elbow positioned next to your ribs. Place the back of your affected hand against the wall. Place a small pillow between your arm and torso.

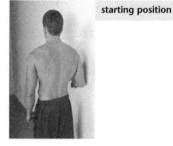

starting position

1 Press the back of your hand into the wall and hold 3–5 seconds. This is a very subtle isometric movement.

VARIATION: This can also be done against a doorframe.

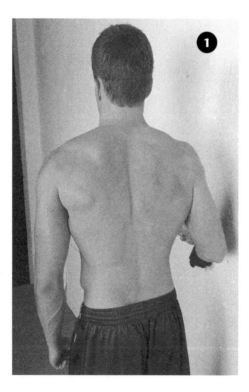

Goal: increase internal rotation strength

STARTING POSITION: Stand facing the edge of a wall or a doorframe. Bend the elbow of your affected arm 90 degrees, keeping your elbow positioned next to your ribs. Place the palm of your hand against the doorframe. Place a small pillow between your arm and torso.

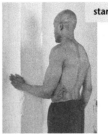
starting position

1 Press your palm into the doorframe and hold 3–5 seconds.

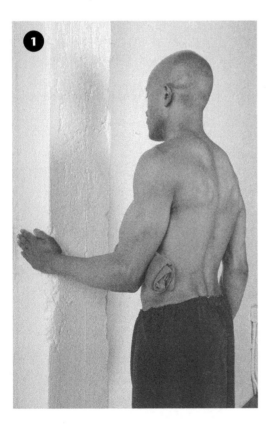

wall push-up

Goal: increase stabilization of shoulder girdle

STARTING POSITION: Stand 2–3 feet away from a wall and place your palms on it, approximately chest height and shoulder-width apart.

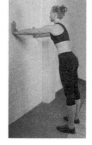

starting position

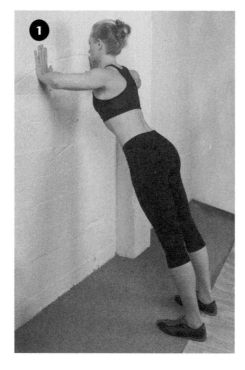

1 Slowly lower your chest towards the wall by bending your elbows. Move slowly and focus on squeezing your shoulder blades together.

Return to starting position very slowly.

VARIATION: To reduce the impact in your shoulders, you can also move just your scapulas, squeezing them together and then expanding them.

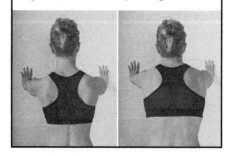

Goal: increase stabilization of shoulder girdle

STARTING POSITION: Stand 2–3 feet away from a wall and place your palms on it, approximately chest height and shoulder-width apart.

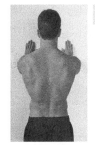

starting position

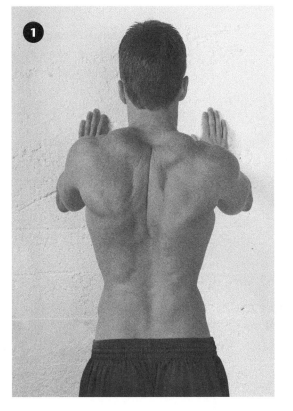

1 Slowly contract/squeeze the muscles between your shoulder blades and hold for 3–5 seconds.

isometric frontal lift
shoulder

Goal: increase shoulder flexion strength

STARTING POSITION: Stand facing a wall and place the back of your affected hand against it.

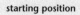

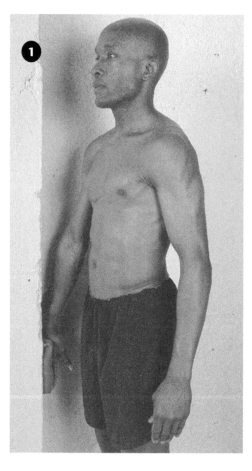

1 Press the back of your hand against the wall. Your arm should be fully extended. Hold for 3–5 seconds, utilizing enough tension to foster muscle tone.

Switch sides and repeat.

Goal: increase shoulder extension strength

STARTING POSITION: Stand with your back to a wall and place the palm of your affected hand against it.

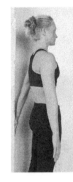

starting position

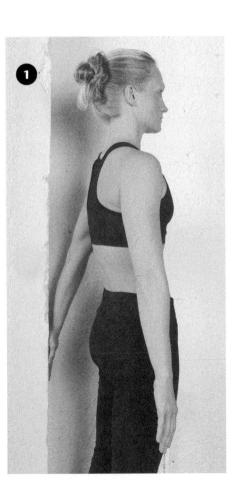

1 Press the palm of your hand against the wall. Hold for 3–5 seconds, utilizing enough tension to foster muscle tone.

Switch sides and repeat.

wall/door series

static pec stretch

chest

Goal: increase shoulder extension strength

STARTING POSITION: Stand against a doorframe or the edge of a wall. Bend your elbow 90 degrees and place your forearm and hand on the wall/doorframe.

starting position

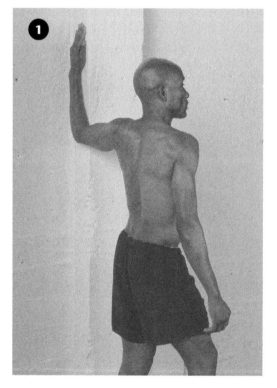

1 Slowly take a step forward, feeling the stretch in your chest.

Switch sides and repeat.

active range of motion series

Each exercise in this advanced series is performed while standing, with focus on range of motion and shoulder blade stabilization. Many of the standing exercises using exercise bands can be performed in a pool. Water exercise provides the advantage of resistance in both directions, and it is difficult to apply too much downward-force load. Once your strength improves, try increasing resistance by using aqua-gloves or hand paddles.

angels   *shoulder*

Goal: increase range of motion and muscle tone

STARTING POSITION: Stand tall with proper posture and your arms at your sides, palms facing forward.

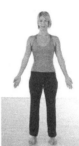

starting position

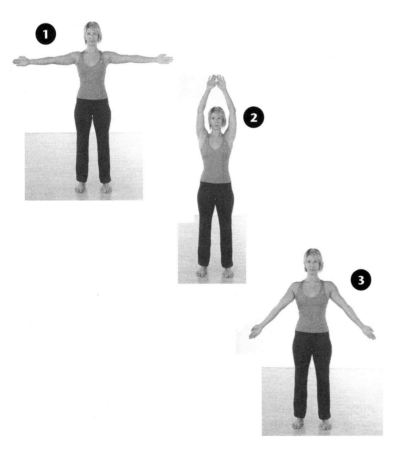

1–2 Inhale deeply through your nose and slowly raise your arms out to the sides as high as comfortably possible. Try to touch your thumbs above your head.

3 Exhale through your mouth and slowly lower your arms.

Repeat as desired.

VARIATION: This can be done one arm at a time.

ADVANCED: Try this movement with your back and arms against a wall.

soup can pours

Goal: increase shoulder flexibility

STARTING POSITION: Stand tall with proper posture and your arms at your side, palms facing backwards.

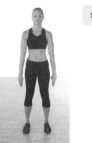

starting position

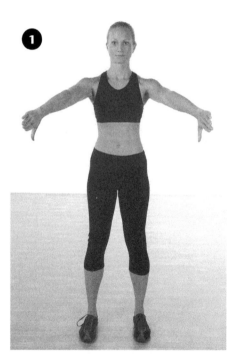

1 Inhale deeply through your nose and bring both arms slightly forward (roughly 45 degrees). As you raise your arms out to the sides, keep your palms facing backwards, actively rotating your thumbs down. Raise your arms no higher than shoulder height.

Exhale through your mouth as you lower your arms.

Repeat as desired.

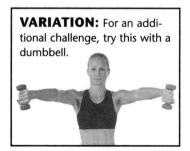

VARIATION: For an additional challenge, try this with a dumbbell.

Goal: strengthen/improve upper back muscles

STARTING POSITION: Stand tall with proper posture and clasp both hands behind your buttocks.

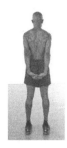

starting position

1 If possible, touch your palms together. Focus on contracting the muscles between your shoulder blades. Do not arch your lower back or allow your neck and head to drop forward. Hold for 3–5 seconds.

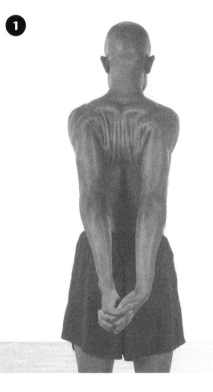

Goal: stretch upper back muscles

STARTING POSITION: Stand tall with proper posture and clasp your hands in front of your body.

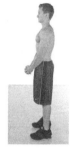

starting position

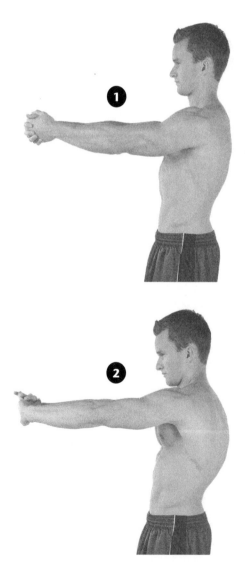

1 Straighten your arms and slowly lift them to shoulder height.

2 Once at approximately shoulder height, turn your palms forward and hold the stretch for 5–15 seconds.

Return to starting position.

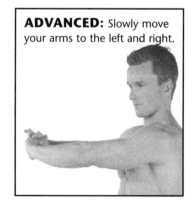

ADVANCED: Slowly move your arms to the left and right.

the wave

Goal: increase range of flexion

STARTING POSITION: Stand tall with proper posture and your arms alongside your body.

starting position

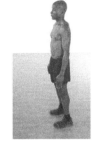

1 Keeping your palms down, raise your arms to a comfortable height, aiming for a complete range of motion.

2 Once at a desired height, slowly lower your arms.

VARIATION: You can also try this with your palms up.

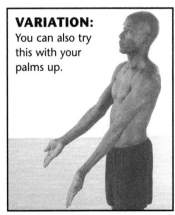

Goal: improve posture and muscles

STARTING POSITION: Stand tall with proper posture. Raise your arms up to shoulder height and bend your elbows 90 degrees so that your fingers point to the ceiling.

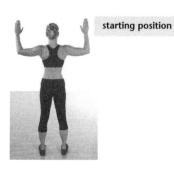

starting position

1

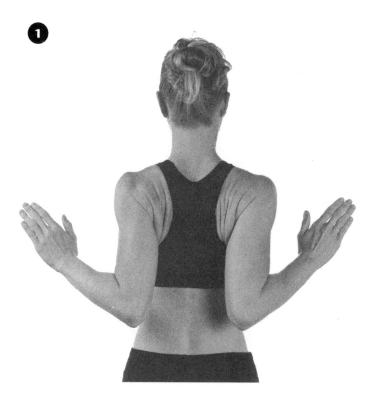

1 Lower your elbows towards your buttocks, as if you're trying to put them in your back pockets. Hold for 5–10 seconds. Do not hold your breath. The purpose of this exercise is to open up your chest and contract the muscles of the upper back, keeping your shoulders back and down.

Goal: increase and improve range of shoulder flexion and functional shoulder movements

STARTING POSITION: Stand tall with proper posture. Clasp your hands in front of your body.

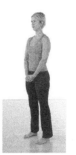

1 Keeping your arms straight, slowly raise them as high as possible. Do not arch your back.

2 Slowly lower your arms to starting position.

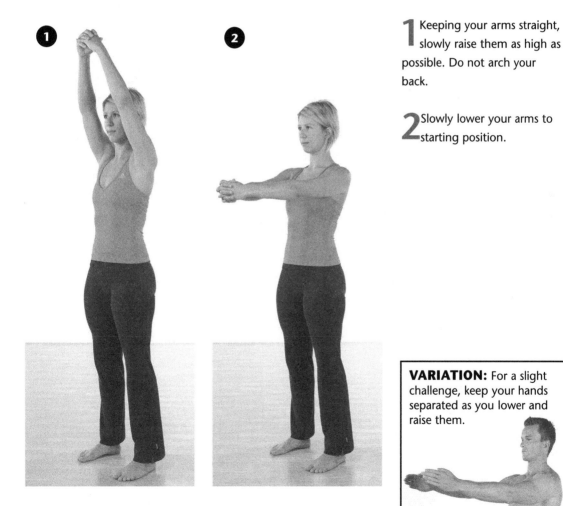

1

2

VARIATION: For a slight challenge, keep your hands separated as you lower and raise them.

118

active range of motion
condor
scapular and humerus joints

Goal: increase range of motion, stabilization and rhythm of the scapular and humerus joint

STARTING POSITION: Stand tall with proper posture.

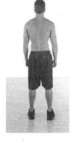

starting position

1

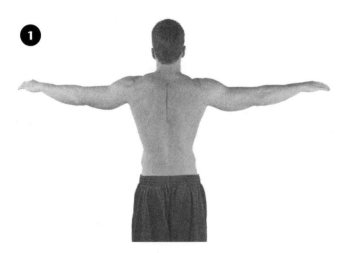

1 Slowly lift your arms to shoulder height and extend your arms out to the sides, keeping your shoulder blades down and inward.

2 Pinch your shoulder blades together.

Slowly lower your arms to starting position.

2

Goal: increase scapular/humerus rhythm

STARTING POSITION: Stand tall with proper posture. Raise both arms out to the sides to make a T shape, palms facing forward.

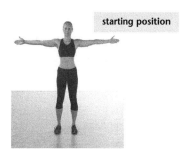

starting position

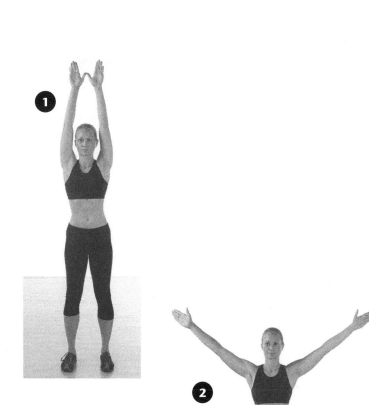

1 From the T position, attempt to keep your shoulder blades down and in "locked position." Raise your arms straight above your head if possible. This resembles the motion of a drowning victim signaling for help.

2 Lower your arms to T position, focusing on shoulder blade placement.

Goal: increase range of flexion

STARTING POSITION: Stand tall with proper posture and your arms alongside your body.

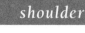

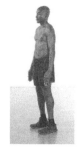

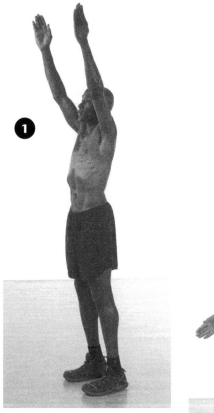

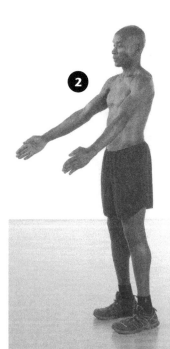

1 Turn your thumbs up while keeping your arms straight, and raise your arms as high as possible.

2 Lower your arms slowly.

VARIATION: Perform the same movement, except focus on keeping your shoulder blades down and in. You'll notice that you have less shoulder flexibility but that is OK.

Goal: increase extension of the shoulder girdle and posterior muscle tone

STARTING POSITION: Stand tall with proper posture and your arms alongside your body.

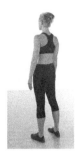

starting position

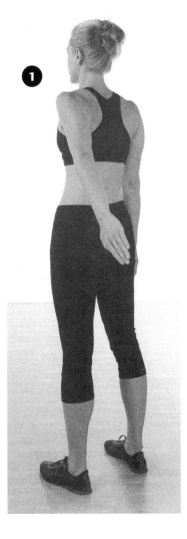

1 Slowly and carefully move one arm back as far as is comfortable. Hold for 3-5 seconds. If you feel pain, do not continue.

Slowly return to starting position and switch sides. Compare the range of motion between your affected arm and unaffected arm.

Goal: increase flexibility

STARTING POSITION: Stand tall with proper posture. Raise your right arm above your head and let your hand drop behind your neck.

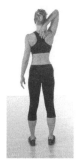

starting position

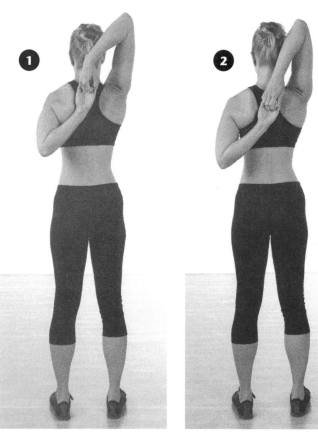

1 Bring your left hand behind your back and clasp the fingers of your right hand.

2 Gently pull down your right hand with your left hand. Hold the position for a comfortable moment.

Switch sides and repeat.

VARIATION: If you cannot reach your hands, use a towel.

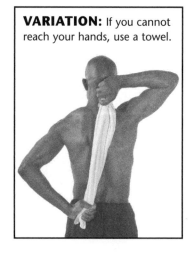

Goal: increase rotator cuff strength

STARTING POSITION: Stand tall with proper posture and your arms at your sides. Squeeze a block or rolled-up towel between your right arm and your torso. Bend your elbow 90 degrees so that your thumb points up.

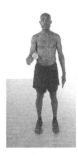

starting position

1

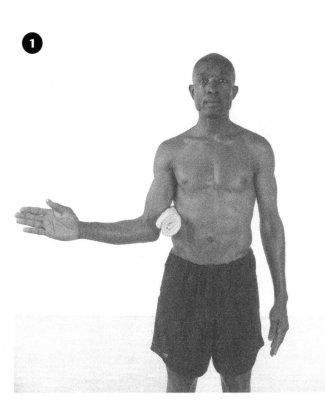

1 Keeping your elbow as close to your body as possible and your forearm parallel to the floor, rotate your forearm out to the side.

Rotate your forearm back in toward your body. Repeat as desired before switching sides.

VARIATION: Try this with your palm facing down or up.

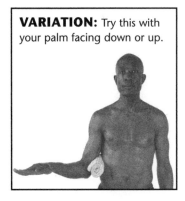

resistance conditioning series

This section utilizes exercise bands or hand-held weights that help improve the strength and muscle tone of the shoulder girdle. When selecting a band, select one that is relatively easy or flexible. Generally, the color of the band denotes the resistance level (e.g., yellow = easiest, red = medium, blue or black = hardest), but not all vendors' bands' resistance levels are equal. When performing strength training for habilitation purposes, do not overstrain your muscles.

Your goal should target proper form and execution. It's important, when using resistance, that you control the movement—don't allow the resistance to control you. Slowly perform the movement in both directions at the same pace (i.e., up, 2,3,4, hold; down, 2,3,4, hold). This will usually prevent further injury.

Hand position and placement is critical when using bands. Grips can be purchased, but this simple device shown below is inexpensive and quite comfortable. (Special thanks to my student Fred Brevold for his idea.) To make a grip, purchase a PVC pipe from any hardware store. You'll also need an exercise band. Once you have both, follow the steps below:

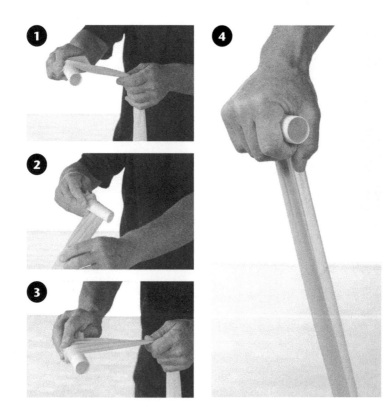

Goal: increase shoulder flexion strength

STARTING POSITION: Stand tall with proper posture. Place one end of the band under the foot on the affected side and grasp the other end with your affected hand. Adjust the resistance by moving your hand up or down the band. Resistance should begin as you start raising your arm. Your arm should be as straight as possible but not locked.

starting position

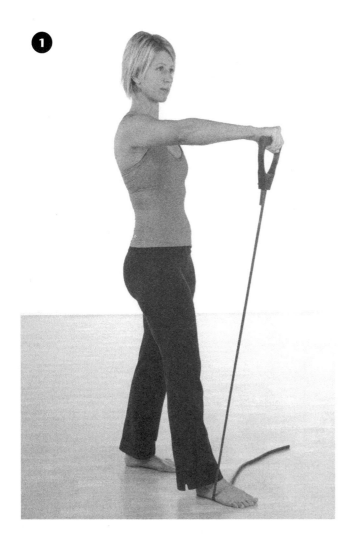

1

1 Slowly bring your straight arm up to shoulder height. If comfortable, raise your arm all the way up. If this is uncomfortable, lower your arm to starting position.

Switch sides and repeat.

VARIATION: This exercise can also be done with dumb-bell weights instead (see page 139).

Goal: increase shoulder abduction strength

STARTING POSITION: Stand tall with proper posture. Place one end of the band under the foot of the affected side and grasp the band with your affected hand, palm down.

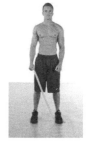
starting position

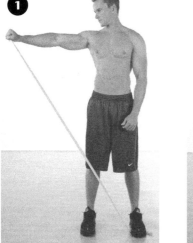

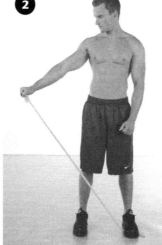

1 Slowly raise your arm out to the side until it's shoulder height. If this is uncomfortable, move the position of your arm to a different angle to find a comfort zone. If this is still uncomfortable, don't do this movement.

2 Slowly return to starting position.

Switch sides and repeat.

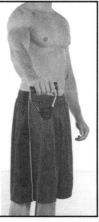

VARIATIONS: If you have trouble lifting your arm laterally, try taking your arm 45 degrees forward.

This exercise can also be done with dumbbell weights instead.

Goal: increase shoulder extension strength

STANDING POSITION: Stand tall with proper posture. Place one end of the band under the foot of the affected side and grasp the band with your affected hand, thumb pointing forward.

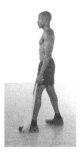

starting position

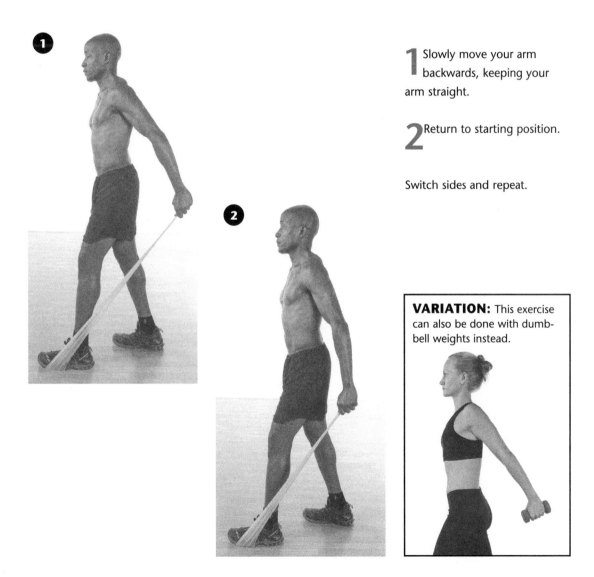

1 Slowly move your arm backwards, keeping your arm straight.

2 Return to starting position.

Switch sides and repeat.

VARIATION: This exercise can also be done with dumbbell weights instead.

T's with band

Goal: strengthen muscles behind the shoulder blades, improve posture, provide stabilization

STARTING POSITION: Stand tall with proper posture. Grasp the exercise band in front of you with your hands shoulder-width apart and palms down. Do not wrap the band around your hands. Keeping your arms straight, raise them to approximately shoulder height.

starting position

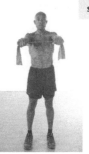

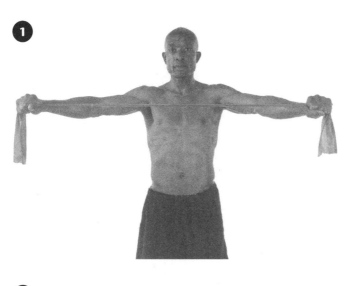

1 Slowly open your arms to the sides, with special focus on squeezing the muscles that bring your should blades together.

2 Slowly return to starting position.

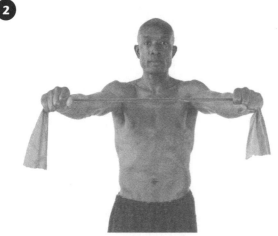

Goal: increase upper shoulder and back strength

STARTING POSITION: Stand tall with proper posture and hold the band with the unaffected hand. Grasp the band with the affected hand at a position that provides mild resistance.

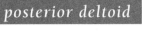

starting position

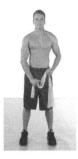

1 Keeping your unaffected arm in place, use your affected hand to pull the band diagonally up and across your body, as if pulling a sword out of its sheath.

Slowly return to starting position. Switch sides and repeat.

Goal: increase rotator cuff strength

STARTING POSITION: Stand tall with proper posture. Grasp the band in both hands with your palms up. Bend both elbows 90 degrees, keeping your elbows next to your ribs.

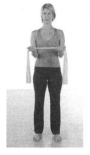
starting position

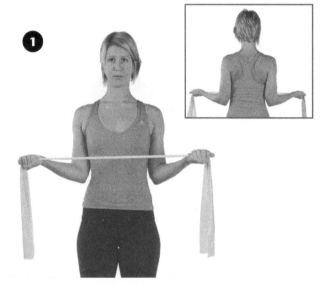

1 Keeping your elbows glued to your ribs, slowly move the ends of the band away from each other as if serving appetizers. Pinch your shoulder blades together. Hold for 3–5 seconds.

Return to starting position.

VARIATION: If you feel any discomfort, try the External Rotation with Band (page 132) or perform the External Rotation (Wall) (page 104).

Goal: increase internal rotation strength

STARTING POSITION: Attach the exercise band to a doorknob or a solid object (such as a heavy table leg), making sure it doesn't come loose. Position your affected side closest to the doorknob. Grasp the band with your affected hand and bend your elbow 90 degrees, placing your elbow next to your ribs. To avoid wrist pain, make sure you grasp the band correctly. You can place a rolled-up towel or small pillow between your elbow and your body.

starting position

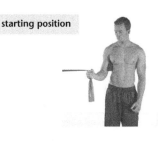

1 Keeping your elbow glued against your ribs, slowly move your hand inward, as if to place your palm on your belly button.

Slowly return to starting position. Switch sides and repeat.

1

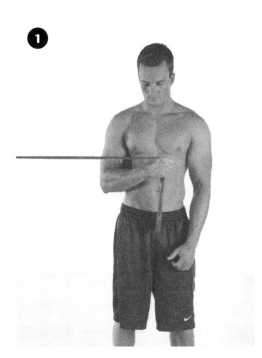

VARIATIONS: If you feel any discomfort, try the Internal Rotation (Door) (page 105).

You can also do this with a partner.

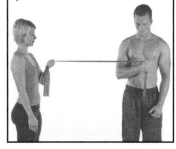

Goal: increase external rotation strength

STARTING POSITION: Attach the exercise band to a doorknob or a solid object (such as a heavy table leg), making sure it doesn't come loose. Position your affected side farthest away from the doorknob. Grasp the band with the affected hand and bend your elbow 90 degrees, placing your elbow next to your ribs. To avoid wrist pain, make sure you grasp the band correctly. You can place a rolled-up towel or small pillow between your elbow and your body.

starting position

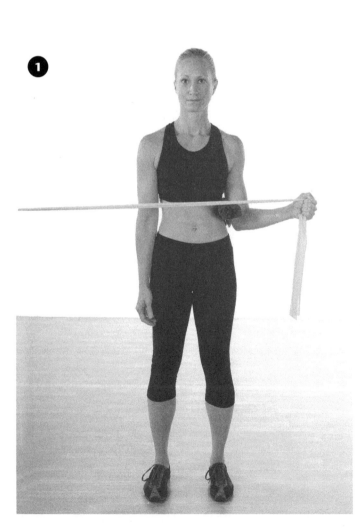

1 Keeping your elbow glued against your ribs, slowly move your hand away from the doorknob, as if opening up a coat.

Slowly return to starting position. Switch sides and repeat.

VARIATIONS: If you feel any discomfort, try the External Rotation (Wall) (page 104).

You can also have a partner hold the other end of the band.

Goal: increase upper back strength

STARTING POSITION: Sit in a chair with proper posture and place a band around the foot of your affected side. Grasp the ends in each hand. Extend the leg straight forward and adjust your hands so that the band offers adequate resistance.

starting position

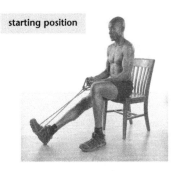

1

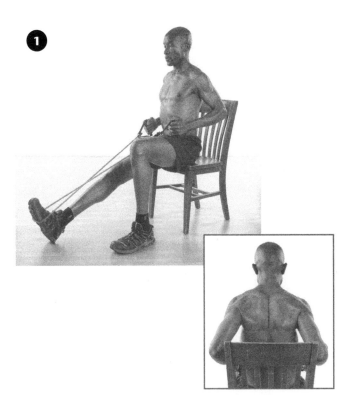

1 Slowly pull the band towards your torso, pulling your shoulder blades together and allowing your elbows to move back.

Slowly return to starting position.

Goal: increase muscle strength between shoulder blades

STARTING POSITION: Secure the band to the top of a door or other high, solid object. Sit in a chair with proper posture. Reach up and grab the ends of the band in each hand, making sure to grasp at a place that offers moderate resistance. Your arms will form a 45-degree angle with the door.

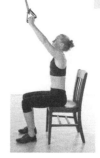

starting position

1 Slowly pull down the band towards your chest, with focus on squeezing the shoulder blades together.

2 Return to starting position while trying to keep your shoulder blades together. Only your arms should move.

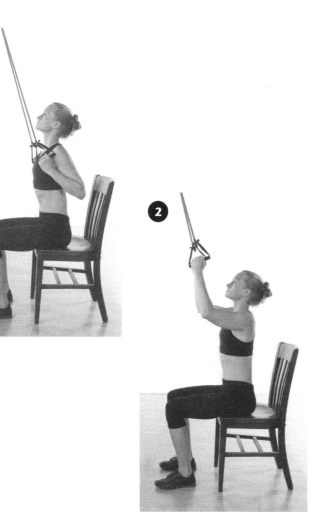

Goal: stabilize shoulder

STARTING POSITION: Stand with proper posture and place the band around your back at chest height. Grasp the ends of the band in each hand at a place that offers moderate resistance.

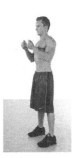

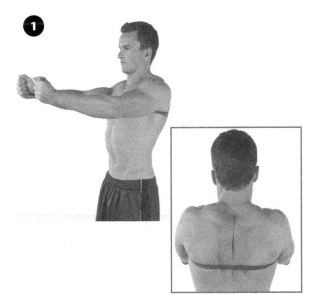

1 Fully extend your arms forward while focusing on keeping your shoulder blades back and stable.

2 Control the motion as your arms return to starting position. Do not allow the band to recoil you.

VARIATION: This can also be done while sitting.

band series

band shoulder press

deltoids

Goal: stabilize shoulder

STARTING POSITION: Sit in a chair with proper posture and place the band around your back and under your armpits. Grasp the ends of the band in each hand at a place that offers moderate resistance.

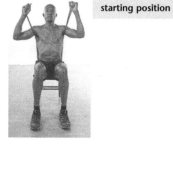

starting position

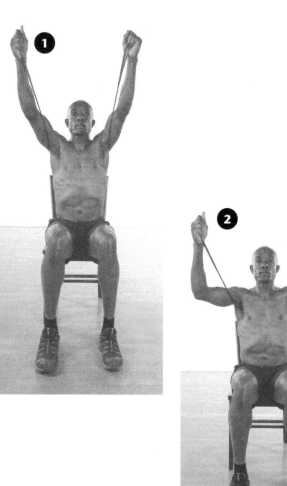

1 Fully extend your arms upward, keeping your shoulder blades together. The amount of upward motion depends on your flexibility and pain tolerance. Some people cannot go directly up and that is OK. Your focus should be on replicating the motion of putting something in an overhead luggage bin, so a slight angle is fine.

2 Control the motion as your arms return to starting position. Do not let the band recoil you.

Y's with band

Goal: increase shoulder girdle strength

STARTING POSITION: Sit in a chair with proper posture and grasp an end of the band in each hand, keeping your hands shoulder-width apart. Raise your arms overhead as high as is comfortable for you.

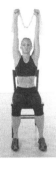

starting position

1 Keeping your head straight and squeezing your shoulder blades together, slowly pull the band apart, forming a Y with your arms.

2 Slowly return to starting position.

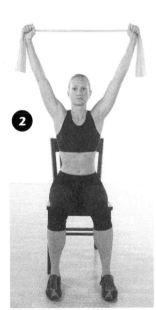

Goal: improve rotation of the shoulder joint

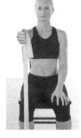
starting position

STARTING POSITION: Sit in a chair with proper posture and hold the end of a band in one hand. Extend your arm forward at shoulder height with your thumb up.

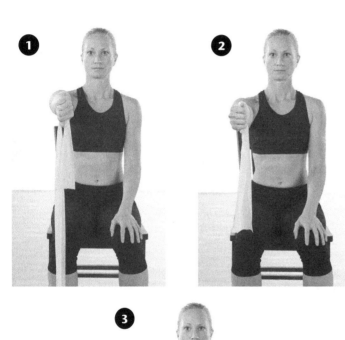

1

2

3

1–3 Turn your hand up and down to collect the band.

Once you've rolled up the band in your hand, switch sides.

dumbbell frontal raises
anterior deltoid

Goal: increase deltoid strength

STARTING POSITION: Stand tall with proper posture and grip a dumbbell with your affected hand. Your arm should be alongside your body.

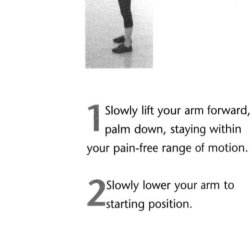

starting position

1 Slowly lift your arm forward, palm down, staying within your pain-free range of motion.

2 Slowly lower your arm to starting position.

Switch sides and repeat.

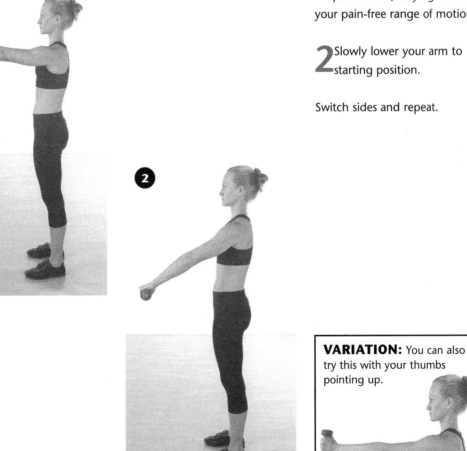

1

2

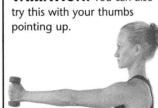

VARIATION: You can also try this with your thumbs pointing up.

dumbbell series

dumbbell shoulder extension

posterior deltoid

Goal: increase rear deltoid strength

STARTING POSITION: Stand tall with proper posture and grip a dumbbell with your affected hand; you can stagger your feet if you need more balance. Your arm should be alongside your body, and your palm can face forward or backward, whichever is most comfortable.

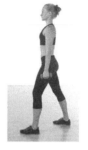

starting position

1 Keeping your arm straight, slowly move it backwards, staying within your pain-free range of motion.

2 Slowly return your arm to starting position.

Switch sides and repeat.

VARIATION: The exercise can also be done lying face down on an incline bench.

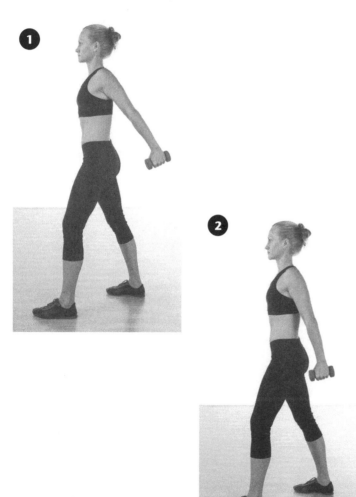

dumbbell soup can pours

Goal: increase shoulder girdle stabilization

STARTING POSITION: Stand tall with proper posture and grip a dumbbell with your affected hand. Turn your thumb down, as if pouring out soda from a can.

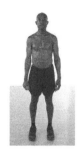

starting position

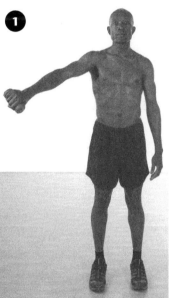

1 Slowly lift your arm out to the side at a 45-degree angle. Focus on keeping your thumb down and not moving your arm forward.

2 Lower slowly, staying within your pain-free range.

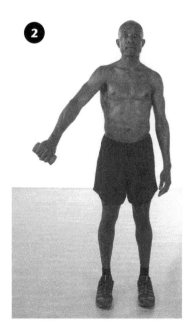

dumbbell series

reverse fly

Goal: increase upper back strength

STARTING POSITION: Lie on your stomach on an exercise bench or bed. Let your affected arm hang off the side. Grip a dumbbell with your affected hand.

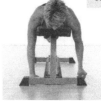

starting position

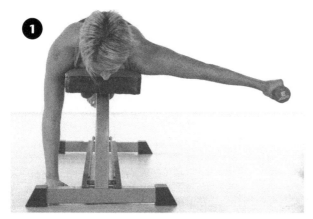

1 Slowly raise your arm to a parallel position with the floor.

2 Slowly return to starting position.

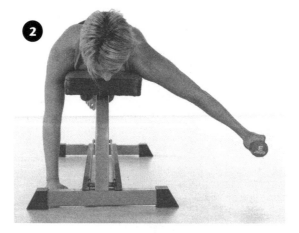

Goal: *increase shoulder girdle control*

STARTING POSITION: Lie on your back on the floor or an exercise bench. Grip a dumbbell with your affected hand and lift your arm directly over your shoulder/chest. Keep your arm straight.

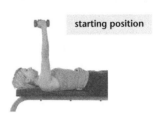

starting position

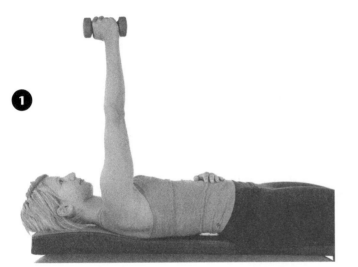

1

1 Keeping your arm straight, press the dumbbell up, as if trying to touch the ceiling.

2 Squeeze your shoulder blades together to return to starting position. The range of motion of this exercise is very small. If your arm is moving frequently, the exercise is not being performed correctly.

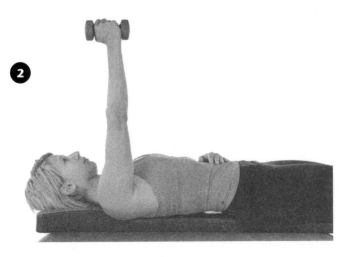

2

dumbbell series

dumbbell shrugs

trapezius

Goal: increase shoulder girdle strength

STARTING POSITION: Stand tall with proper posture and your arms along your sides. Hold a dumbbell in each hand.

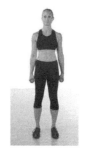

starting position

1

2

1–2 Shrug your shoulders up and then back, squeezing your shoulder blades together. Pretend you are making an outline of a box.

Slowly lower your shoulders to starting position.

hanging dumbbell squeeze

Goal: increase upper body strength, traction and stabilization

STARTING POSITION: Place your right knee and hand on an exercise bench. Grip a dumbbell with your left hand and allow the weight to pull down gently on your arm. Do not use a heavy dumbbell.

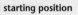

starting position

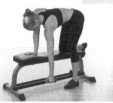

1 Keeping your arm straight, gently squeeze your shoulder blade up and back to pull the weight up. Hold for 3-5 seconds.

Slowly release and lower.

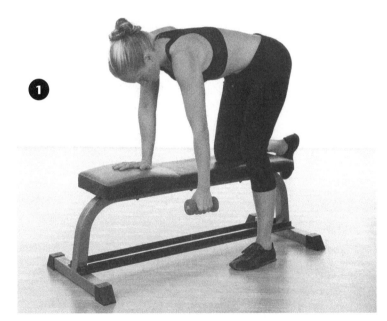

dumbbell series

prone crossing guard

rotator cuff

Goal: increase strength of rotator cuff

STARTING POSITION: Lie on your stomach on a bed or an exercise bench with your affected arm hanging off the edge. Grip a dumbbell and bend your arm 90 degrees.

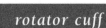
starting position

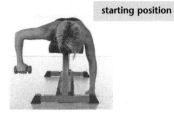

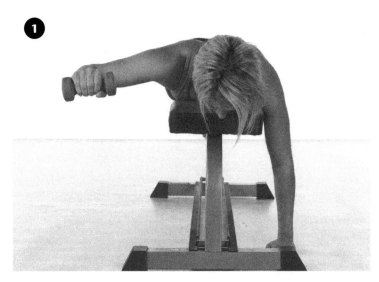

1 Keeping your elbow in place, slowly rotate your hand up to the ceiling. STOP when your hand is level with your shoulder. Many people are inflexible in this area and have limited range of motion. If you feel any discomfort, skip this exercise.

Lower your arm to starting position.

VARIATION: You can also try this with both arms simultaneously.

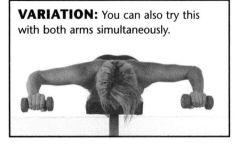

self-massage

Performing self-massage or gently squeezing the shoulder area can prepare the joint for motion or provide relief after an exercise/therapy session. It decreases soft tissue adhesions, increasing range of motion and flexibility. It also decreases muscle soreness. Self-massage is best performed when the muscle is warm. Here we use the standard tennis ball as well as the commercially available foam roller, which can be purchased online and at various local retailers, including medical suppliers, yoga/Pilates studios, and sporting goods stores.

tennis ball method 1   *upper back, shoulder*

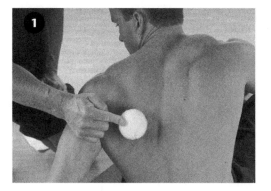

1–3 With a single tennis ball, lie on your back, placing the tennis ball under the point of discomfort to release pressure.

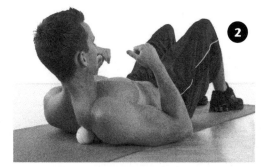

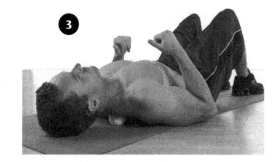

self-massage

tennis ball method 2

upper back, shoulder

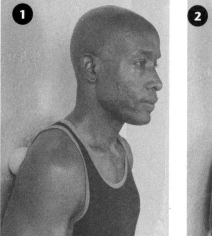
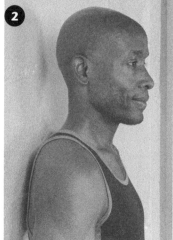

1–2 Place a tennis ball between your back and a wall and roll around to release pressure.

tennis ball method 3

latissimus dorsi

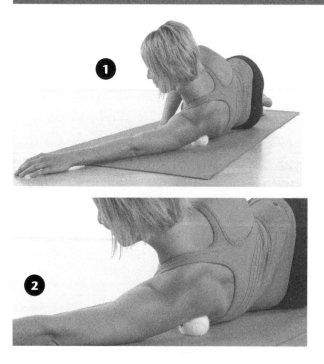

1–2 To target tight lats, lie on your side and place the tennis ball under your armpit. Roll around to release tightness.

tennis ball method 4   *chest, shoulder*

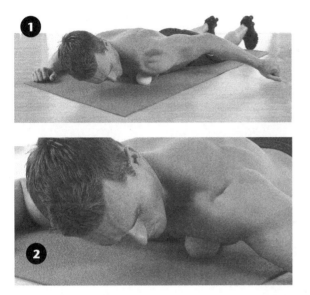

1–2 To target the front of your shoulder, lie on your front, placing the tennis ball under the point of discomfort to release pressure.

tennis ball method 5   *chest, shoulder*

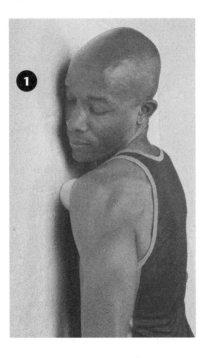

1 Place a tennis ball between the front of your shoulder and a wall and roll around to release tension.

self-massage

tennis ball method 6 — *upper back*

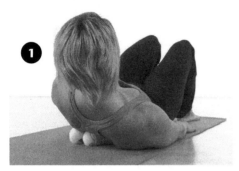

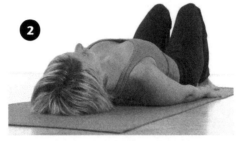

1–2 Connect two tennis balls together with tape so that they look like googly eyes. Lie on them so that they're between your shoulder blades.

tennis ball method 7 — *upper back*

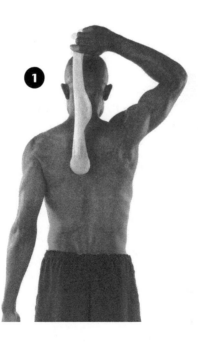

The nice thing about the sock is that you can more easily target those awkward areas of the back.

1 Take an athletic sock and place 1 or 2 tennis balls inside it. Reach the sock overhead and let it hang behind your back. Press your back and the balls against the wall, releasing tension.

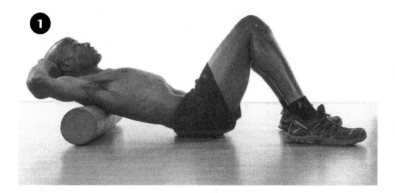

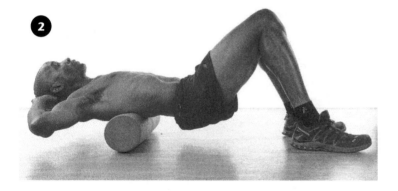

1 Sit on the floor and place your upper back on a foam roller. Clasp your hands behind your head.

2 Roll back and forth to release tension.

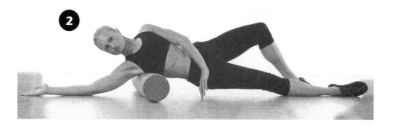

1 Lie on your side with the foam roller under your armpit.

2–3 Roll back and forth to release tension.

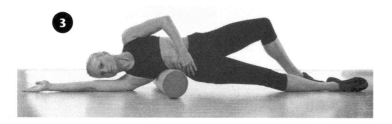

To create the cooling massage tool, place water in a paper cup and freeze it. An ice massage is best done after exercise.

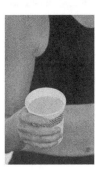

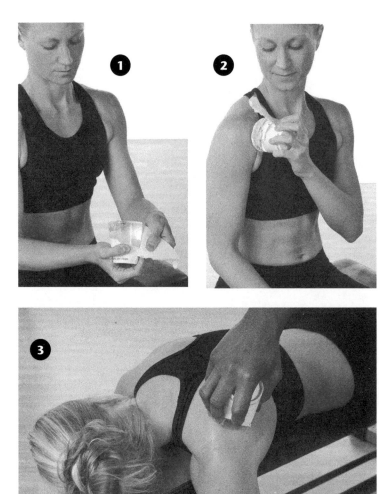

1 Peel back the paper cup as needed.

2 Apply the cup of ice on the sore spot, moving the cup around—do not leave it on one spot.

3 Ask a partner to get the hard-to-reach places.

resources

American Academy of Orthopedic Surgeons
6300 North River Road
Rosemont, IL 60018
(847) 823-7186
www.aaos.org

American Board of Orthopaedic Surgery
400 Silver Cedar Court
Chapel Hill, NC 27514
(919) 929-7103
www.abos.org

American Chronic Pain Association
P.O. Box 850
Rocklin, CA 95677
(800) 533-3231
www.theacpa.org

American Physical Therapy Association
1111 North Fairfax Street
Alexandria, VA 22314
(800) 999-2782
www.apta.org

index

other books from karl knopf

Healthy Hips Handbook: Exercises for Treating and Preventing Common Hip Joint Injuries
$14.95
Healthy Hips Handbook is designed to help prevent hip problems for some and, for those with existing hip problems, provide post-rehabilitation exercises.

Core Strength for 50+: A Customized Program for Safely Toning Ab, Back and Oblique Muscles
$15.95
Core Strength for 50+ has everything you need to improve posture, enhance sports performance, guarantee low back health and avoid injury.

Foam Roller Workbook: Illustrated Step-by-Step Guide to Stretching, Strengthening and Rehabilitative Techniques
$14.95
Details a comprehensive program for using the foam roller to recover from injury, reverse everyday pain and stay healthy in the future.

Kettlebells for 50+: Safe and Customized Programs for Building and Toning Every Muscle
$14.95
Provides sport-specific workouts that allow aging athletes to maintain the flexibility, strength and speed needed to win.

Make the Pool Your Gym: No-Impact Water Workouts for Getting Fit, Building Strength and Rehabbing from Injury
$14.95
Shows how to create an effective and efficient water workout that can build strength, improve cardiovascular fitness and burn calories.

Stretching for 50+: A Customized Program for Increasing Flexibility, Avoiding Injury and Enjoying an Active Lifestyle
$14.95
This book shows the 50+ individual how to maintain and improve flexibility by incorporating stretching into one's life. Specially designed programs cater to every fitness level.

Total Sports Conditioning for Athletes 50+: Workouts for Staying at the Top of Your Game
$14.95
Provides sport-specific workouts that allow aging athletes to maintain the flexibility, strength and speed needed to win.

Weights for 50+: Building Strength, Staying Healthy and Enjoying an Active Lifestyle
$14.95
Weight training is one of the most effective ways to get healthy and fight the physical signs of aging. *Weights for 50+* shows how easy it is for anyone to get started with weights.

To order these books call 800-377-2542 or 510-601-8301, fax 510-601-8307, e-mail ulysses@ ulyssespress.com, or write to Ulysses Press, P.O. Box 3440, Berkeley, CA 94703. All retail orders are shipped free of charge. California residents must include sales tax. Allow two to three weeks for delivery.

acknowledgments

It is a joy to work with such a team of professionals, without whose skill and expertise this book would not have been possible. I would like to sincerely thank Lily Chou, Rupa Ved and Claire Chun, whose attention to detail and ability to explain complex concepts in user-friendly terms is without parallel. Thanks also to models Samuel Harvell, Scott Mathison, Meredith Miller and Bernadett Otterbein for their patience, and to Austin Forbord and his team at Rapt Productions, who were able to capture the essence of the exercises so well. I'd like to thank acquisitions editor Keith Reigert for his vision. Lastly, a special note of appreciation to two people who served as my fact checkers: Dr. Fiona Gilbert and my son Chris Knopf.

about the author

KARL KNOPF, author of *Stretching for 50+*, *Weights for 50+* and *Total Sports Conditioning for Athletes 50+*, has been involved with the health and fitness of the disabled and older adults for 30 years. A consultant on numerous National Institutes of Health grants, Knopf has served as advisor to the PBS exercise series "Sit and Be Fit," and to the State of California on disabilities issues. He is a frequent speaker at conferences and has written several textbooks and articles. Knopf is president of Baby Boomers & Beyond (www.babyboomersandbeyond.net). He also coordinates the Fitness Therapist Program at Foothill College in Los Altos Hills, California.